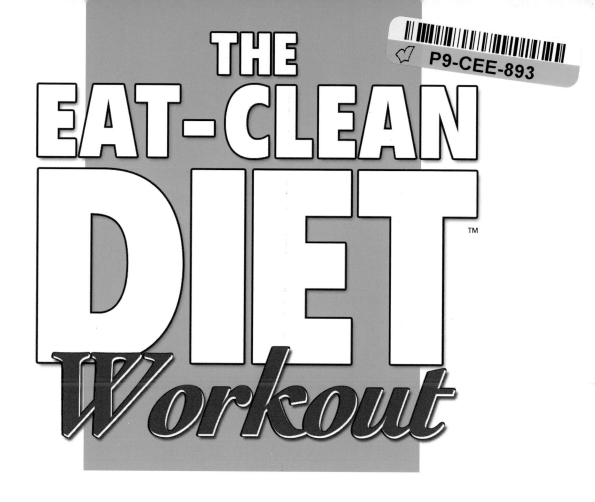

THE
EAT-CLEAN
DIET ™
Workout

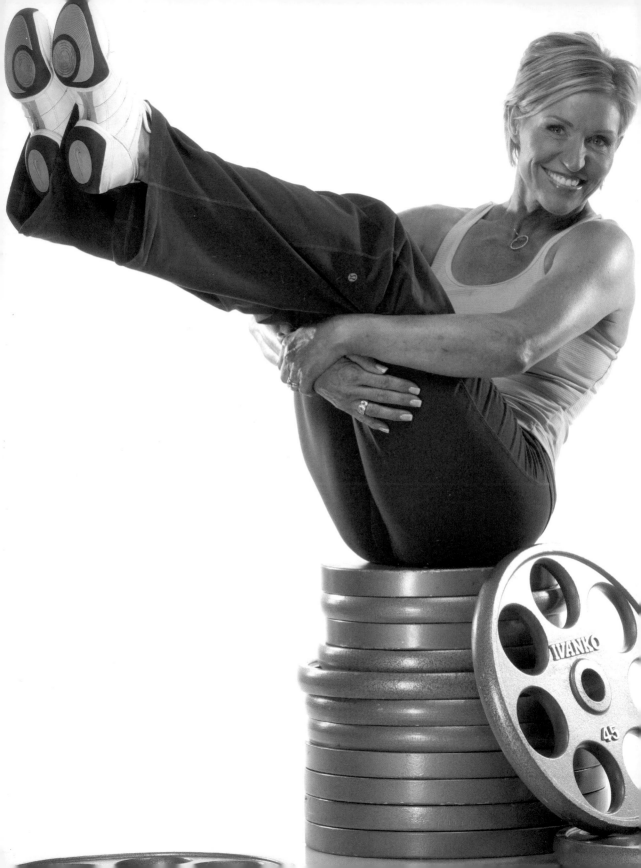

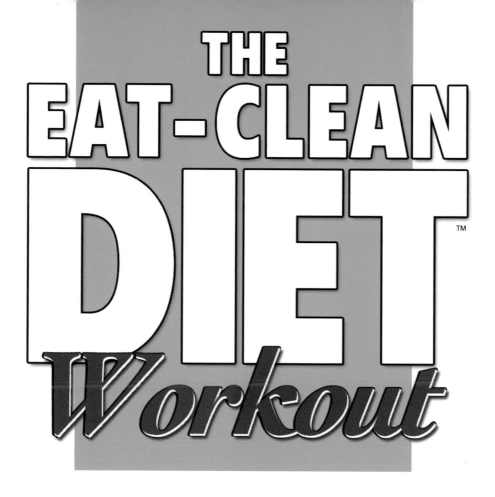

THE EAT-CLEAN DIET™ Workout

Quick Routines for Your Best Body Ever!

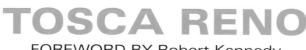

TOSCA RENO

FOREWORD BY Robert Kennedy

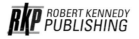

RKP ROBERT KENNEDY PUBLISHING

Published by Robert Kennedy Publishing
5775 McLaughlin Road
Mississauga, ON
L5R 3P7 Canada
Visit us at **www.eatcleandiet.com**

Design by Gabriella Caruso Marques
Edited by Wendy Morley and Rachel Corradetti

National Library of Canada Cataloguing in Publication

Reno, Tosca, 1959-
          The Eat-Clean Diet Workout : Quick Routines For Your Best Body Ever! / Tosca Reno;
foreword by Robert Kennedy.

ISBN-13: 978-1-55210-045-5
ISBN-10: 1-55210-045-6

          1. Stretching exercises. 2. Cardiovascular fitness. 3. Weight training for women.
      4. Physcial fitness for women. I. Title.

RA781.6.R46 2008   613.7'045   C2007-906151-6

10 9 8 7 6 5 4 3 2 1

Distributed in Canada by
NBN (National Book Network)
67 Mowat Avenue, Suite 241
Toronto, ON
M6K 3E3

Distributed in USA by
NBN (National Book Network)
15200 NBN Way
Blue Ridge Summit, PA
17214

Printed in Canada

IMPORTANT

The information in this book reflects the author's experiences and opinions and is not intended to replace medical advice.

Before beginning this or any nutritional or exercise regimen, consult your physician to be sure it is appropriate for you. Ask for a physical stress test.

Dedicated to the Sisters in Iron: You will become one the moment you lift your first weight.

I also dedicate this to my family for supporting all that I do.

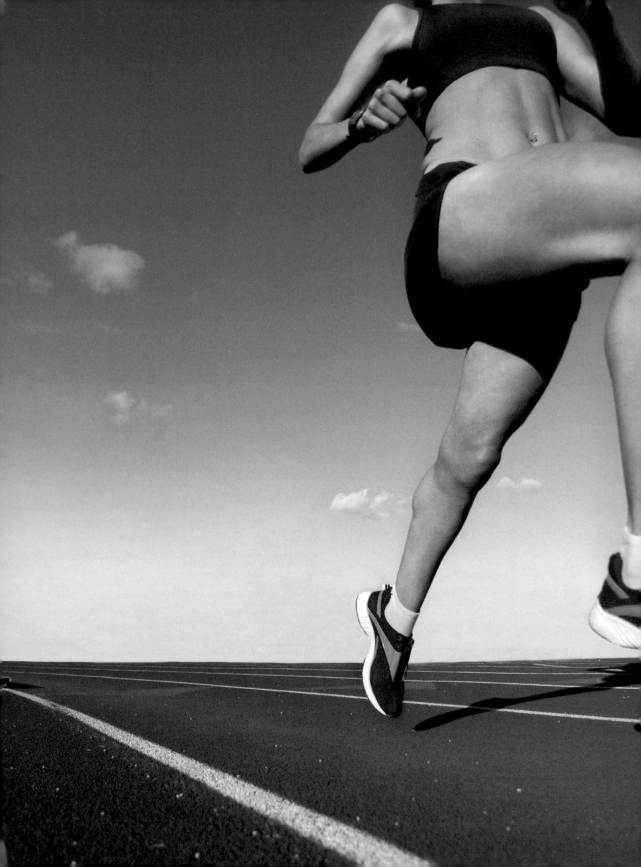

CONTENTS

FOREWORD

I am in the business of body shaping, and through the years I have seen much. Every so often a phenomenon comes along that makes me wonder how I managed without it. Think television, cell phones and personal computers in the technical world. Then think dumbells, treadmills and aerobics classes in the fitness world. Now here comes a gal who combines the essentials of Clean Eating, striking good looks (even for a woman nearer 50 than 40) and iron-willed determination towards weight training. Suddenly everyone is looking at body shaping with different eyes. How did we manage without Tosca Reno?

I call it the pop-out effect. When you see Tosca, you suddenly get what the fuss is all about. She stands out from black print and white paper with a clarity and vitality that arrests you right where you stand. The runaway success of her book *The Eat-Clean Diet* ensured she was on the radar of North Americans hungry for a new, healthy way of eating that would help them shed pounds and improve their quality of health and life. The "Clean Eating" term went viral. Everyone's talking about it.

Now she's done it again. With her Beautiful Body Formula: 80% nutrition + 10% training + 10% genetics

"Fat or thin, tall or short, young or not so young, you can change your physique and enjoy a brand new healthy lifestyle."

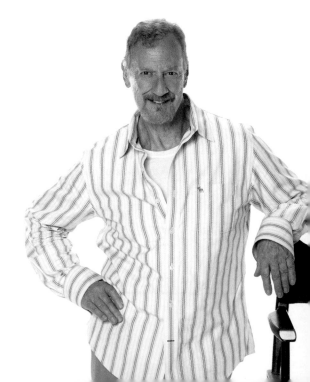

Reno stresses the significance of nutrition in achieving an ideal physique. In *The Eat-Clean Diet Workout*, Reno tells the rest of the story. Training, in her eyes, is not just about building a lean, muscular body. It is also about fortifying the emotional self, especially one that has had a few hard knocks, as we all have. When life handed her the worst and crisis seemed imminent, Reno got up off the couch and picked up the iron. As she states: "With every weight I lift and every rep I do, I am rebuilding my self-esteem. I have never felt stronger and more confident. Whereas I used to slink into a room and hope no one would notice, I now take my place in the world because I have something to offer. I want others to experience this too."

The Eat-Clean Diet Workout is a never-been-done education of weight training that embraces both the novice and the pro. Weights are the tools of choice and Reno is the teacher who walks the walk and talks the talk. She relates to the Newbie who has never lifted a weight, guides her along the journey of learning to lift and celebrates the appearance of her first muscular curves. For the experienced lifter she offers challenging training programs that will cut up, rip up, define and dazzle.

Reno's feisty style is a refreshing change to so much pap spooned out to a population deserving of much more. Never before has the need for her fervent counsel been so urgent as we face not only a North American obesity epidemic but now a global one. Today, our children face the very real possibility that they will not live the long healthy lives their parents did, thanks to inferior nutrition and its devastating dancing partners diabetes, heart disease, cancer and stroke. Thankfully, Reno has come along to gently but firmly coax us back onto the right path.

If you ever thought there was no hope, stop thinking that right now. Take Reno's example as yours. Starting at age 40 she turned her life around with the help of Clean Eating and a serious love affair with weight training. Don't accept that it's too late. Let the phenomenon that is Tosca Reno, with her longed-for practical approach, inspire you to become your own best self. Once you do you won't know how you ever managed without her. You'll see. This book is written for you.

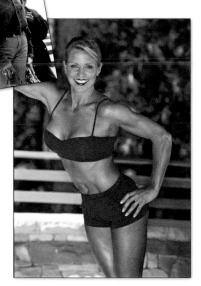

◄ BEFORE, age 40.

Publisher of Oxygen Magazine

INTRODUCTION

Believe it! You can use weights to sculpt your body in the same way a sculptor uses a mallet and chisel to create a work of art. Simply visualize the way you have always wanted your body to look, and get to work! Add a little here – take some off there. Lose weight, gain weight. Shape up, slim down, add muscle and lose fat. Whatever it takes, the fitness way of life is the answer and it will do the job faster and more healthfully than any other method known to women anywhere.

The beauty of weights is that you can tailor the resistance to your condition. In other words, if you are excessively thin and weak, you can start by using extremely light weights to slowly ease yourself into shape. As you tone up, lose fat and improve your shape, you will be able to add a little more weight to the bar. Gradually, with patience and dedication, you will accomplish your dream: your optimal condition of health and physical appearance.

Remember, you are in charge of the weights. They are the tools with which you can sculpt your body to physical perfection. Use them according to my recommendations and the benefits will amaze you in the same way they have amazed me. For the last eight years and counting I have been successful at keeping a lean physique through the combined efforts of weight training and Clean Eating. I have not been disappointed.

Weights are often referred to as iron pills. Today's doctors, scientists, personal trainers, coaches and educators are in agreement about the enormous advantages gained from regular usage of resistance-training equipment. If weights *were* pills, they would be known as magic pills – those that so many

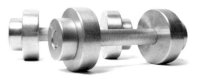

of us have been chasing since the obesity epidemic has overtaken North America. The benefits gained through their regular use are little short of miraculous. Eight years ago I had excess weight to lose – over 70 pounds! Clean Eating slimmed my body down while weight training rearranged the flats to curves. I was hooked from the word "Go!"

Tailored for You

Do you have any reservations about the current women's fitness look? You know, the woman with

TIP

This was the most eye-opening experience — that you could actually shape your own body.

ripped hardcore muscles and attitude to match. I will say my first experience seeing such lean-muscled women intimidated me, too! I thought, 'How could I ever look like that? There is surely no hope for me.' But once you get the idea that training manifests magnificent bodies it doesn't take much persuasion to give it your best shot. We are all Sisters in Iron once we pick up the weights – whatever the number on the side!

I have heard the question many times. "You wouldn't want to look like a musclehead, would you?" When a question like that comes around it always seems to me the questioner really means: "Don't you agree that women who display that kind of muscularity look awful? They look mannish. Even ugly!"

You can admire such a physique without wanting to emulate it, just as you can be a fan of gymnastics without wanting to train like a gymnast. There is something powerful and confident about these women with muscle that I wanted to taste. As a young mother I had traded away much of my power to "others." A body that exuded confidence was just what I needed. With every weight I lifted I became not only physically stronger, but also mentally and emotionally whole.

When you first see a competitive fitness woman you could find the experience strange. If you are not used to seeing muscular women with low body-fat levels, you may think it looks unnatural. When you get used to seeing superior female physiques you

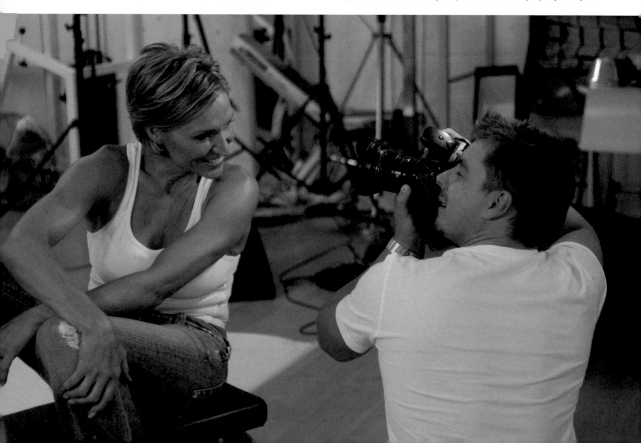

will come to realize the true beauty of a completely trained feminine body. No sport builds and shapes a woman's body as perfectly as weight training. When runway models are compared with the likes of top figure athletes such as Monica Brant, Alicia Marie, Jennifer Nicole Lee or Mary Elizabeth Lado, it's "No contest!" When it comes to physical beauty, the trained fitness woman wins hands down.

Body of Art

Individuals will differ greatly in their skeletal proportions and aptitude for adding muscle. Different women have wide or slim hips, narrow or wide shoulders, long or short legs. But scientific training, as explained in this book, can help you harden up, balance out, and look and feel dynamic – more dynamic than you have ever looked or felt in your life. The stage may not be your goal and stacks of muscle may not be in keeping with your goals either, but a lean layer of muscle on any physique will help you stand out from the crowd and become a head turner in your community. Your doc will love the training too, since you cannot fail to improve your overall health.

There is no such thing as the perfect physique. But if you are serious about sculpting your body, your dedication will get you as near to perfection as humanly possible. I have seen many physiques and faces that are not in the purest sense beautiful, but with training and a captivating smile the most ordinary person becomes stunning. Don't allow anything to prevent you from becoming your best you!

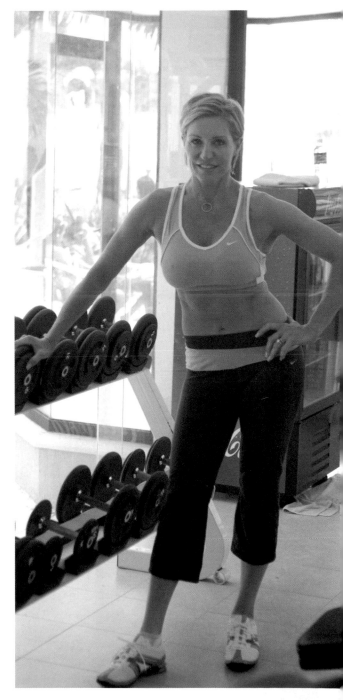

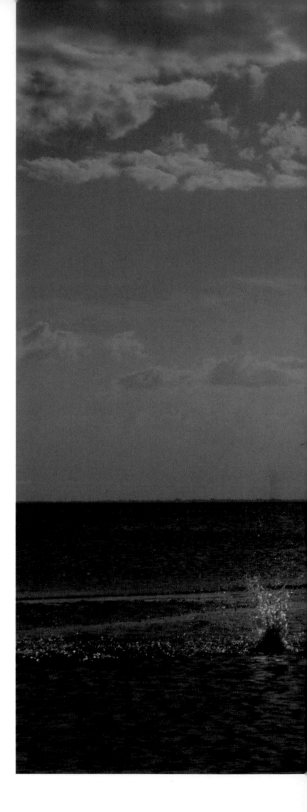

If you are not yet convinced of the beauty of women's fitness, look again. Study the pictures in this book. Above all, remember this: You don't have to be big. I certainly am not and have no wish to be. I competed in bodybuilding once. I loved the experience but learned early on I don't have a bodybuilder's body. Remember, you are in control. You decide what is enough or too much muscle for you. Develop your body to the degree you wish. Just wait for that exhilarating moment when your jeans become loose at the waist and your blouse buttons up with no strain across the chest. Then you will get your first compliment and you will surely be hooked.

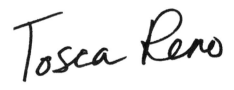

I did not start out with a perfect body. Far from it! With over 70 pounds of excess fat and an exhausted state of mind I was at my worst. Start there, start anywhere, but do begin. It will be the start of a magical transformation.

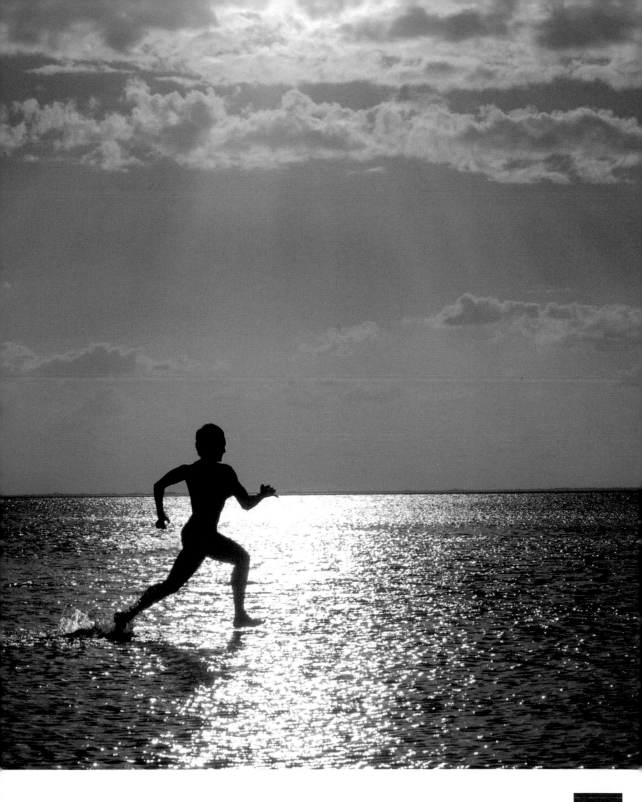

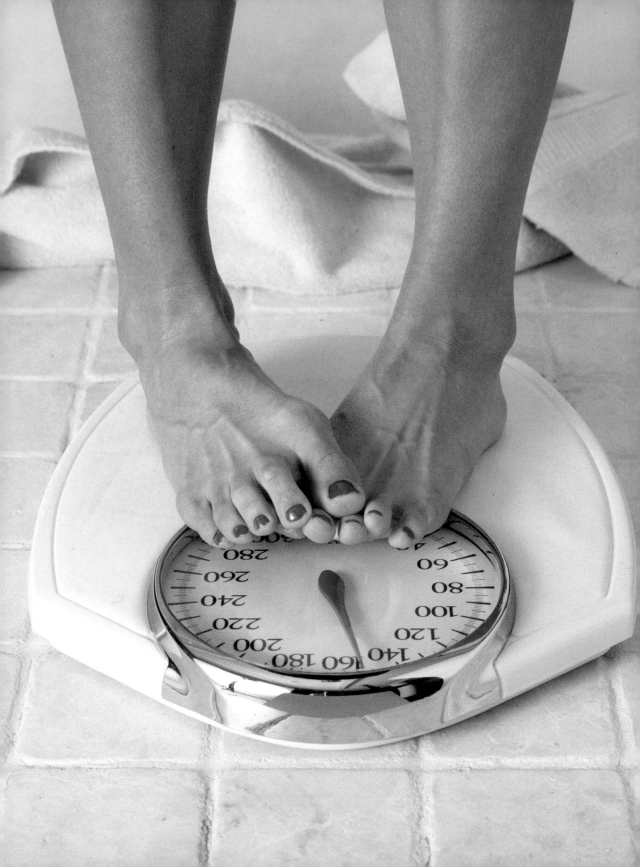

1

CHECKING OUT YOUR BODY
CRITICAL EVALUATION

Self-evaluation is an important part of body shaping because it gives you a base from which to work. As the sculptor has to start with an unshaped piece of wood or stone, you must begin with the shape your body is in right now. That means you have to ask yourself some tough questions. How fit are you? How fat are you? Are you underweight? Are you healthy? Are you happy with where you are right now?

The surest way of finding out if you have too much fat under your skin is to try the pinch test (medically known as the skinfold test).

We all have to go through this drill if we want to change. I did it. My weight was so out of control I couldn't decipher if I was hungry or full and ate for all the wrong reasons. I could hardly climb up the steep steps of my Victorian home without having to stop and catch my breath. I measured and weighed myself, pulled out the Fat Pictures and got comfortable with the idea that this was going to have to change. Now!

If you are in doubt about your present appearance, try the mirror test. Take all your clothes off and stand in front of a full-length mirror. Turn on all the lights. Do this at a time when you are completely alone.

You don't want any distractions. Cast your eyes across your shoulders. Look at your arms, chest, and waistline. Take in your hips, thighs, and calves. Check your overall proportions. Are your calves big enough? Have you too much weight on the upper thigh area? Is there fat around your belly and lower back? Are your upper arms much thicker near the shoulders than they are near the elbows? Now try to decide what you want to correct. Is your posture good? Are you carrying excess weight? How much? Do you need to put *on* weight?

The surest way of finding out if you have too much fat under your skin is to try the pinch test (medically known as the skinfold test). Simply pinch some of your skin between your thumb and forefinger. The best sites are the triceps (back of the upper arm), side of the waist, top of outer thigh, and side of chest. If your pinched skin is more than half an inch, this is an indication that you are carrying too much fat.

Another method of assessing your current weight and physical condition is the Waist-to-Hip ratio. This measurement takes into account the circumference of your waist and compares it to the fullest part of your hips. The resulting number predicts your fat distribution and whether or not you are at a greater risk for certain disease. The world over, the ideal Waist-to-Hip ratio is considered 0.7:1, but anything under 0.8:1 is considered healthy.

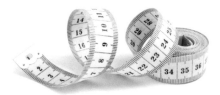

TOP WAYS TO MEASURE
BODY COMPOSITION

CALIPER/SKINFOLD TESTS

Accurately measures the subcutaneous fat on the body. Devices called calipers are used to grab a double fold of skin and adipose tissue from up to nine sites on the body. The sum of the skinfolds is calculated and applied to equations to determine body-fat percentage. Does not consider visceral adipose tissue.

1

2

WAIST-TO-HIP RATIO

An accurate and simple test whereby waist and hip girth are determined with a measuring tape. Waist girth is divided by hip girth to determine a ratio. Values below 0.85 for men and 0.80 for women are acceptable. A strong relationship has been found between waist and hip relativity and heart disease.

HYDRODENSITOMETRY (UNDERWATER WEIGHING)

Accurate test measuring the density of the body under the premise that muscle weighs more than fat and will cause the body to be more dense. The more dense the body the more it will weigh underwater.

3

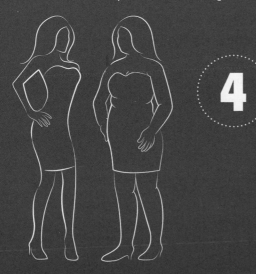

4

BIOELECTRICAL IMPEDANCE (BIA)

Accurate test measuring the conductance of an electrical current through the body. Specific conductivities are known of fat mass and fat-free mass in the body. Therefore, the composition of the body can be computed.

DUAL X-RAY ABSORPTIOMETRY (DEXA)

Very accurate test whereby two X-rays measure the body's mineral mass, fat mass, and fat-free mass. The amount of X-ray photon absorbed by the mass is directly proportional to the amount of tissue present.

MAGNETIC RESONANCE IMAGING (MRI):

Very accurate but expensive technique used to excite water and fat molecules using a magnetic field. The reading given by the excited molecules shows how fat is distributed throughout the body.

AIR DISPLACEMENT PLETHYSMOGRAPHY (BOD POD)

Accurate but expensive test similar to underwater weighing. This technique uses the displacement of air to determine the density of the body.

BODY MASS INDEX (BMI)

A common but inaccurate test using an individual's height and weight to determine body mass. It does not take into account that muscle mass weighs more than fat mass. Hence, a lean bodybuilder could have a greater BMI than an obese individual.

COMPUTED TOPOGRAPHY

Accurate but expensive test used to take cross-sectional scans of the body. It provides an image of the body and is best used to determine intraabdominal fat versus subcutaneous fat distributions.

Taking Stock

Excessive fat obscures shape. It fills in areas where one muscle curves into another. It replaces the natural arc running from the waist to the hips. It shrouds the descending silhouette from the hips to the knees. Fat on the upper outer thigh creates a bulge where a smooth curve would otherwise be. The knees, together with the ankles and wrists, should always be bony and virtually devoid of fat, thereby emphasizing the curves of the thigh and calf muscles. Superfluous fat in the knee and ankle area will give your leg a straight, unattractive appearance.

We have created many names for these fatty deposits, including Muffin Top, which is the fat spilling over the top of your pants, Cankles for a thick calf that descends down into a thick ankle, Bat Wings for flabby triceps, the Wattle for the hanging flesh under your throat, Buddha or beer belly for a round tummy, and Thunder Thighs for heavy legs.

One way of determining how you look is to have someone take a few digital pictures of your body. You will be able to immediately scrutinize your physical condition. Compare these with pictures from when you felt you looked your best. The important thing is that you become totally aware of your shape. Learn about yourself. Try to determine what your ideal weight should be. Is a particular body part troubling you?

Maintain a level of awareness about your physical appearance and half the battle is won. You have to know where you have been to know where you are going.

This experience of assessing your physical self need not be a damaging experience. It will be if you focus on everything that's "wrong" with you. But if you do that you will never progress. Rather, harness positive energy around the fact that you are sitting here with this book in your hands, wanting very much to make healthful changes to your body for YOUR OWN reasons. When the spirit of change is driven by your desire to improve, no one will be able to stop you. Make this about you and taking care of you.

When the spirit of change is driven by your desire to improve, no one will be able to stop you.

Fitness Level

It may be harder to evaluate your physical fitness. No one wants to admit they are out of shape and everyone thinks they can do more than they can. If you can run up a few flights of stairs without being seriously out of breath, then you are probably fit. On the other hand, if you feel bad after walking a block or two, then you are not in the shape you thought you were. But don't worry. This book is for everyone and everyone has to start somewhere, just as I did.

Whatever your current fitness level, I strongly recommend that you ask your doctor to give you a physical stress test. Tell him or her the type of exercise you will be doing. By all means show your doctor this book. It is always advisable before undertaking any new type of exercise or nutrition program to have a complete medical checkup. You will find that a stress test can be fun (you will probably have to step up and down on some boxes or jog on a machine while your breathing and pulse are monitored). After you get the go-ahead from your doctor, you'll be

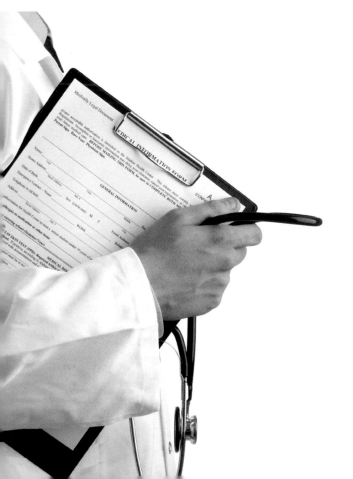

thrilled that you have a clean bill of health. Alternatively, should an irregularity be uncovered, you're still ahead, because you can take steps to improve your health. Again, this is your starting point. There is no reason to stop your efforts before you have even left the gate. Nearly everyone – not just the sublimely coordinated – can weight train. However, it can pose a problem to those with heart or circulatory disorders such as high blood pressure or other organic malfunctions, so be sure to check with your doctor if in doubt. I can't stress that enough!

Whatever you do, resist the temptation to suddenly throw yourself into endless furious sessions of formal exercise. Remember, I am going to help you coax, not pound, your body into a new dynamic shape. I do not want you to be hindered by unnecessary aches and pains. Your new body will certainly develop – but do the job right and follow the steps.

The Age Factor

Men usually discover weights between the ages of 16 and 19. The reason is simple. They are tired of being skinny and laughed at, or their football coach tells them not to show up for practice unless they get into shape. Women, on the other hand, often start to exercise only when they see deterioration in their condition. They suddenly realize that their clothes don't fit or they are no longer comfortable wearing certain items – particularly body-revealing items like swimsuits. Thousands of men also take up training to lose flab, of course, and untold numbers of skinny women want to add flesh to their limbs. However, most ladies undertake a program of formal exercise to lose excess fat and to tone up their bodies.

Many of these women will be asking these questions: Is it too late? Am I too old? I have been asked these questions not just by people from their 50s to 70s, but also by people in their 20s and 30s. Even teens! Somehow folks think they need to be athletic and young to train, and that is just not true.

The truth is, you can start training at any age. Just follow the advice of this book carefully and tailor the exercises to your present condition and needs. The urge to get into shape can hit you at any stage in life; age does not automatically disqualify you. I am very relieved to have discovered this, otherwise I may never have started.

Throw Out the Scale

One of the nicest things about exercise is that it erases your fear of the bathroom scale. Women have dieted for ages, basing their evaluation of the body on scales, instruments designed to measure pounds *only*, not the difference between the body's muscle and fat content. If you are not already aware of it, muscle weighs more than fat. This means that you can actually weigh more while losing fat because you are adding muscle as the fat is discarded. Essentially you are exchanging lighter (yet bulkier) fatty tissue for denser, toned muscle tissue. In the end you will be leaner and healthier, with less fat and more muscle.

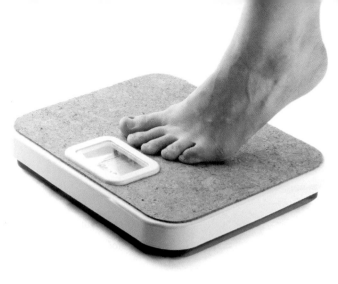

Women who work out seldom worry about what the scales say. It's the mirror that counts. A body is judged by its shape, not by its weight!

Once you have carefully evaluated your present condition, then develop what *Oxygen* publisher Robert Kennedy calls "clear vision." Set your goals realistically and map out your journey to success. Clear vision means: Translating your needs and desires into reality without wasting energy on anxiety, without constantly asking, "Am I doing the right thing?" Don't allow negative influences to destroy your dreams of physical perfection or superstardom. Your dream can be reality, as I discovered.

A body is judged by its shape, not by its weight!

Facts and Fiction

Whereas a woman's progress in the fitness arena does not equal, or very seldom equals, that of a man, neither do women have to achieve as much as men. The average man may weigh 150 pounds with 12-inch arms and a 38-inch chest. To become a bodybuilder he would have to increase those statistics to approximately a 250-pound body weight, 19-inch arms, and a 50-inch chest.

In modern competition, even at the highest level, little benefit is gained by a woman who has arms bigger than 12 inches. Far from wanting to build their bodies, most female newcomers to weight training actually want to become smaller. Women also understand how much resistance training can do for strengthening the skeleton, especially in the face of advancing age and fears of osteoporosis. They find weight training seems to "turn back the clock."

A Better Life

So what can you expect from regular exercise with weights? According to Joyce Vedral, Ph.D., "By following the fitness lifestyle, you can quickly and efficiently improve your appearance, health, physical fitness, mental outlook, and your sex appeal."

Working with weights increases endurance and flexibility and improves your heart and lung functions. Dr. Nagler, Physiatrist-in-Chief at the Cornell Medical Center in New York City, offers another plus: "As women get older, they tend to stoop at the shoulders. Weight training helps them maintain an erect posture for a much longer time by keeping the back extensor muscles strong."

"By following the fitness lifestyle, you can quickly and efficiently improve your appearance, health, physical fitness, mental outlook, and your sex appeal."

A study published in *The Physician and Sportsmedicine* magazine indicates that female athletes who train with weights are three times less likely to be injured in sports-related activities. If injuries do occur, weight trainers recuperate twice as quickly as the control group. The reasons? Stronger muscles and tendons guard against injury. Greater overall strength gives more support to the other parts of the body and helps you withstand abuse. The study also reported that female trainers are "somewhat less anxious, neurotic, depressed, angry, and confused, and more vigorous, extroverted, and self-motivated than the general population." These are just some of the excellent reasons you might want to pursue weight training.

Muscle Myths

Naturally you will come up against muscle myths, the most common one being that weight training will turn you into a muscle-bound freak. This is just not true. When it comes to building man-sized biceps, women don't have enough of what it takes: namely, man-sized levels of testosterone, the male hormone responsible for muscle growth. Unless you have above-average amounts of this hormone and only if you are prone to general hulkiness, you'll never be mistaken for Arnold Schwarzenegger's sister. Progressive exercise will lead to improved muscle tone, and with high-intensity workouts you will increase your muscle size to a degree. However, you will add only limited size while reducing body-fat percentage, resulting in the coveted "toned" look.

True or False?
Weight training will turn you into a muscle-bound freak.

False!

There's nothing to be afraid of when you take up weight training. There are no undesirable side effects from progressive resistance exercise. It is a healthy pursuit, and one that complements other pastimes. Vigorous exercise helps your mind function at its best and conditions you for other sports and activites – even the demanding game of life.

The fitness way of living is captivating because the well-being and appearance-enhancing factors are undeniable. Aren't you excited to read on? This book will reveal the wonders of pumping iron – something I had no idea about when I first started years ago and now could not envision my life without. I will show you exactly how to completely remold your body to a new dynamic shape. Your best life is ready to be lived.

GETTING STARTED
Controlled Ambition

Every day hundreds, perhaps thousands, of women begin weight training. If you are a beginner, there is one thing I know for sure: You are confused! I know this because I had absolutely zero clue about weight training when I started, and that was most intimidating for me. I can imagine what you may be feeling right now. If you can get past the fear you will make it, I promise.

Fitness training is not an exact science. Not only will you read of different rules for resistance exercises, you may well see opposing views printed in the same magazine. Believe me, I have seen it! The most rigid opinions are often held by those with the least knowledge. While there is always room for different ideas and opinions, I suggest that you stick to my advice in the beginning. Once you have a solid understanding of the basics of weight training and are in tune with your own body, you can try some new and different concepts.

Basics for Beginners

There are basic dos and don'ts for resistance training. These give you the best chance for success. If you are like me at all, you may be tempted to skip this section, but if you can hold out you may reach your physique renovation destination faster. So here we go …

Beginners seek the fastest, surest, and safest way to lose fat, build lean muscle, gain strength, have vigorous health, and achieve well-being. High on the list is fat loss. Often Newbies go at it on their own or by taking bad advice from anyone who happens to be standing nearby. The result? Their training progress is slowed or nonexistent and they end up tired and

disenchanted with the whole scene. Frustrated, they often give up.

Remember, the shortest route to success is the correct route, and that means embracing some simple rules. If you choose the wrong path at the beginning of your journey, you may never get to your destination. Picture a ladder placed against a wall – any wall – and climbing as if your life depended on it. When you reach the top you realize you were climbing the wrong ladder. You were climbing like mad, but you did not get where you wanted to go. Avoid wasted effort by doing it right in the first place, even if this means going slowly.

Fitness training for the beginner must be simple. There's no shame in simple. Your first steps as a baby were not sure or steady but eventually you were running. Your training should involve workouts that are relatively short to allow sufficient recuperative time for the broken-down muscle tissue to repair itself. When you lift a single weight over your head you break down trillions of cells. It is the continual breaking down and building up of cells that causes you to build lean muscle mass. To do this properly you must also Eat Clean regularly and get adequate sleep.

Sleep Easy

So there you have it: exercise, food and rest. Get them right and you are on your way! You will notice that rest is hardly a problem once you incorporate

TIP

Want to look better, faster? Sleep! Your body recovers from all your hard work while you are nestled in your bed. No sleep = no six-pack!

regular resistance exercise into your life. At the end of your busy day you feel a happy tired and sleep comes very easily. Exercise is a wonderful sleep inducer. I believe the feel-good component of weight training is responsible

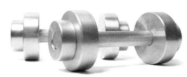

strong and well conditioned right this minute, use only the bar or very light dumbell during the first workout. Picture yourself lifting just the bar and being all right with that. In time, as you gain strength, you will add some weight in almost all of your

What you carve out of your body with weight training will only make you more feminine.

for this, but scientists say it is your body's way of ensuring repair and recuperation, as repair takes place when you sleep.

exercises, but for now go easy and remind yourself you are training with weights and that's a good thing. A very good thing.

Single-Minded Sessions

My initial training sessions were decidedly single minded. I didn't want to embarrass myself. It took all my concentration to get through my first shoulder-press exercise. But my determination was so strong I forgot what was going on around me and put my mind completely into pushing the dumbells above my shoulders. Remember that your session is all about you – not the other guy. Take my words to the gym with you and let them carry you through your training sessions day by day. I am with you all the way.

Training with weights is the most concentrated form of exercise known. Your first few workouts should be performed with very light weights as you grow accustomed to them. This is not a reflection of your inability or lack of strength. Unless you are naturally

Sets and Reps

Sets and reps (repetitions) are two words you need to know, because they are the fundamental terminology of weight training. Over and over you will hear these words. Although they are second nature to me now I remember being very confused about these terms in the beginning. Hearing the phrase: "Perform 3 sets of 10 to 12 reps," for the first time sounded foreign and intimidating. What did it mean?

When you complete an entire movement from start to finish – for example, lifting and lowering a barbell in a barbell curl – you perform one rep. If you complete the movement 12 times before setting the weight down, than you have performed one set of 12 reps. If you pick the barbell up and do 12 more reps, than you have performed 2 sets of 12 reps, or 2 x 12.

Gradual Progression

Beginners should do only one set of each exercise. After a short period (about 10 to 14 days) you can graduate to 2 sets per exercise and soon after that (another couple of months) you may find yourself wanting to do 3 sets per exercise. Pretty soon you will be doing sets and reps as if they were second nature to you. Believe me, it won't take long to learn.

Beginners should not push their bodies to the maximum by rushing from one set of a particular exercise straight into the next set. In general you should move on to the next set when your breathing has returned to normal and your body has settled down from the previous set. In heavy exercises, such as squats, you will require a longer rest period (a few minutes) than you would between less strenuous exercises (30 to 90 seconds). When you progressively decrease the amount of rest you take between sets, you place more stress on the muscles over a shorter period of time. This creates additional intensity. I do this when I am pressed for time and know I won't be able to do both weight training and cardio in the same day. I go into the gym with the idea that I will cut my rest time to as little as 30 seconds between sets and look forward to the intensity of that workout. You also get aerobic benefit from increasing your workout pace. This helps to burn more calories and reduce body fat. Try this when you need a change or when you feel strong enough to have progressed to this stage, about six weeks into your training.

Correct Breathing

Deliberate, forceful breathing during exercise is important and serves several functions. It supplies your entire body with essential oxygen. Without deep breathing you could run out of air, get dizzy, and lose concentration. You could even faint. If you have ever felt that slightly scary, fuzzy feeling during a workout, you may have to adjust your breathing. I have trained many folks who seem to forget all about breathing while they train. I have to remind them that

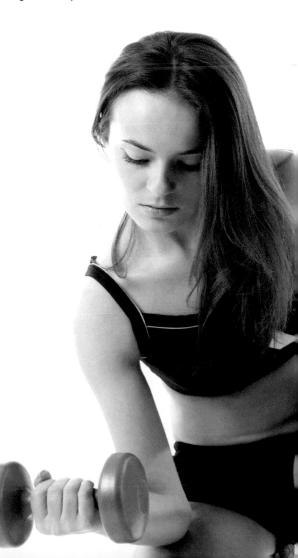

I need to hear them breathing otherwise I worry they may pass out on me.

Regular breathing enables you to use more weight in your exercises and helps you focus on the performance of the movements. It gives your exercises cadence and rhythm, which are other important aspects of successful weight training. In most exercises you should inhale quickly during the easiest part of an exercise and exhale just as the hardest part is accomplished. I like to make a practice of breathing in rhythm with my repetitions. I make a game of it in my head, which helps me count and breathe effectively. However you do it, just remember to breathe and you'll be all right.

Aerobic Exercise

This specific form of exercise depends on the body's use of oxygen. Aerobic exercise, or cardio, is used to condition your organs and circulatory system – the lungs and heart in particular – and is an important aspect of maintaining a healthy heart. Every health-minded woman should practice some form of cardio. Millions of words have been written on the subject, but simply put, aerobic exercise is the repetition of an ongoing movement, such as swimming, rowing, hill climbing, walking, cycling, cross-country skiing, skating, or jogging, for a period of at least 20 minutes, whereby your heart rate is elevated but does not exceed 80 percent of your maximum heart rate.

**To figure out your maximum target heart rate, subtract your age from 220.

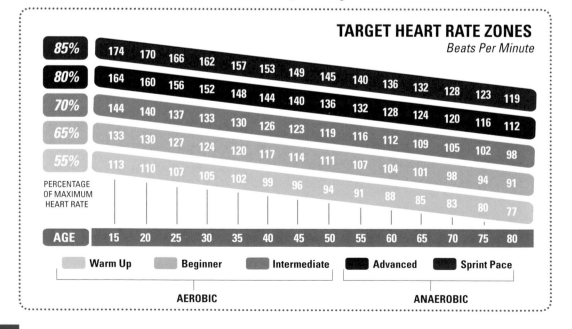

Most treadmills have an interval-training option. You can also use the manual option and adjust the speed yourself.

Aerobic exercise contributes to low body-fat levels. We should all make an effort to incorporate it into our training regimen. Cardio is an important adjunct to weight training, for health and fitness purposes. Those of you trying to gain weight will want to stick to three low-intensity cardio sessions each week. If you are trying to lose body fat, then do up to five or six cardio sessions each week, and make sure your intensity level is high. Be cautious if you are a beginner – push yourself but don't kill yourself.

I love to ramp it up by doing HIITs – High Intensity Interval Training. You break your cardio session into short bursts of high-intensity followed by short periods of the same activity performed at a much lower intensity. Watch the sweat drip from your forehead!

Workout Frequency

Controversy abounds regarding workout frequency. In truth, optimal frequency depends on your level of experience, your tolerance for vigorous exercise, and your ability to recuperate after workouts.

But why lock yourself into training a certain number of times each week? If you choose to train every other day, you would be training four times one week and three times the next. That would work! In general, you should train each body part at least twice

DIFFERENT SPLIT OPTIONS

	SUNDAY	MONDAY	TUESDAY	WEDNESDAY	THURSDAY	FRIDAY	SATURDAY
OPTION 1		Chest Back Arms	Shoulders Legs Abs		Chest Back Arms	Shoulders Legs Abs	

	SUNDAY	MONDAY	TUESDAY	WEDNESDAY	THURSDAY	FRIDAY	SATURDAY
OPTION 2	Chest Back Arms Abs Shoulders		Quads Hamstrings Calves Glutes		Chest Back Arms Abs Shoulders		Quads Hamstrings Calves Glutes

	SUNDAY	MONDAY	TUESDAY	WEDNESDAY	THURSDAY	FRIDAY	SATURDAY
OPTION 3	Chest Back Arms	Quads Hamstrings Calves	Glutes Shoulders Abs		Chest Back Arms	Quads Hamstrings Calves	Glutes Shoulders Abs

and no more than three times weekly. This is the training pattern I follow and I find it most successful.

A good beginner's workout routine is to train your whole body in one workout, three times a week: for instance, Monday, Wednesday, and Friday. A day's rest from the weights following your workout day is necessary for proper muscle recuperation, so schedule a rest day after each weight workout. Do not think you will do yourself any favors by going great guns and taking no day of rest. The only result you will realize is a flat, stringy body and extreme fatigue. If you overtrain or injure yourself at the beginning, you've set yourself up for failure.

The alternative, especially if you have been training for a few months, is to split your routine, performing the first half on one day and the second half the next day. This could translate as training your chest, back, and arms one day, and shoulders, legs, and abdominals the next. You could do upper body one day and lower body the next. Or you could do "pushing" exercises one day and "pulling" exercises the next. You may still take a complete rest day after each workout *(known as the every-other-day split)* or you can work out two days in a row and rest on the third day, then work out another two days and rest the following day, and so on. You will soon learn what works best for you and that will become your workout routine.

Some very experienced women work out even more frequently than this, training three days on, one day off. This is not for beginners. Work your way up to this over an extended period of time. In the meantime, be happy knowing you are doing resistance training – something you may never have done before – and are taking back your life! I am proud of you.

Exercise Performance

The way you perform an exercise is important for your physical safety and serves to keep your muscles in good condition. Actually, most women have a natural aptitude for good exercise style, unlike men, who often forsake good style in the quest to lift additional weight. It's a lot like the man who gets lost but refuses to stop the car and ask for help. His wife would simply pull over and ask, saving a lot of time and trouble.

The golden rule for beginners is to start with light weights and build up gradually. *You* are the best judge of the amount of weight to use for each movement. Stay well within your strength ability. Lifting the "correct" amount of weight for you should feel safe and always as if you are in control. If you are staggering or struggling under a weight, it is too much. Stop immediately and choose a lighter weight.

You should never be so engrossed in lifting a weight that you bend backwards, twist to one side, lift your hips, or swing your body. These are all "cheating" movements. They may help you complete a repetition, but you will be using momentum instead of strength and will succeed only in cheating your muscles out of their proper exercise. You may even injure yourself unnecessarily.

A curl, for example, is for the biceps. When you swing your body back and forth to rock the weight

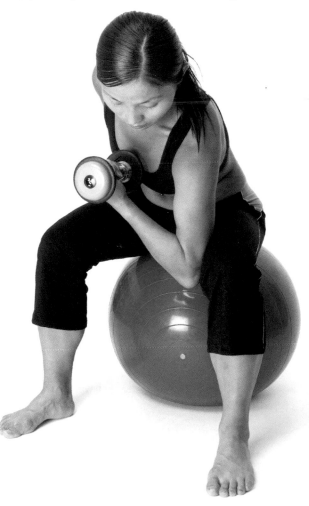

up, you relieve the arms of direct stress because the back and legs aid in the lift. It won't feel right and your biceps won't get any benefit or "sweet pain." For the moment, as a beginner, keep your exercise style strict. Each movement at this stage should involve a complete contraction and extension of the muscles being exercised. Stretch the muscle fully on presses, rows and arm exercises. Rise completely up and down on toe raises, leg extensions, and leg curls. The sooner you learn correct style and form when training with weights the sooner progress will come your way.

Take pride in making each exercise work your muscles over their fullest range. Think about what you look like as you work out. Use a mirror to help ensure that you raise the bar evenly. Constantly check that the dumbells are lifted to the same height and that your body does not twist and contort itself. If you have to contort your body and struggle with the weight it is too much. Perfect exercise style can lead to a perfect physique.

When to Train

The most important consideration about making the commitment to train is that you have given yourself permission to take care of your health, body and well-being. For many women this is the place where the real magic begins. Once you have made this giant leap in your thinking you can and will accomplish anything, and send that positive message to your loved ones at the same time. Good for you!

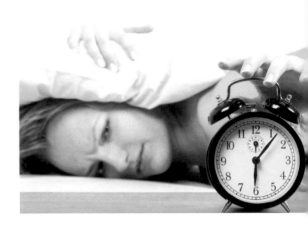

Exactly when to train is up to your own personal timetable. It's a matter of when you can best fit your training in with your work and family commitments. There is some evidence showing that women over 35 have more energy in the early morning whereas

> **If you choose an exercise time because studies show it should be the best, but never make it because that time is inappropriate for your schedule, you'll never benefit.**

younger women have peak energy in the early evening. However, if you choose a time because studies show it should be the best, but never make it because that time is inappropriate for your schedule, you'll never benefit. It's best if you can manage to work out at the same time each day. This will set your internal clock and prepare you for regular training. After a few weeks your body will actually begin to *energize* itself in anticipation of the accustomed training.

At this moment you may be totally "gung ho" on training. If you are, then great! I am all for you. I want you to succeed and become my sister in iron. But over-enthusiasm can be your enemy – it can wipe you out. Take it easy at first. Hold back on your temptation to give it your all. Do the exercises correctly, using the proper style and amount of weight for perfect form. Be satisfied and proud of your efforts to do so. Take comfort in knowing you are building an excellent foundation for your beautiful future.

Flexibility – Stretch It Out

Flexibility is the limberness of joints and muscles that permits a maximum degree of movement. It is made possible by the regular practice of stretching exercises. Stretching is an excellent way of preparing the muscles for training. It also helps keep your joints, ligaments, tendons and muscles flexible. Besides, it is satisfying in itself! Today many women improve their flexibility with regular yoga classes. Numerous recent studies have shown that the more flexible a person remains the healthier she is, even late in life, and the fewer injuries she sustains. This may help explain the current explosion in the popularity of yoga as Baby Boomers flock to classes.

Weight training builds up muscle and tendon strength, but only minimally increases the suppleness of joints, muscles or tendons. Stretching helps keep the joints loose and allows for complete range

TIP

Never bounce when stretching. The point is to elongate the muscle slowly over time, not tear it! Go as far as you can while feeling a gentle pull in the stretched muscle. Never go to the point at which you feel pain. Hold each stretch for 20 to 30 seconds, and remember to stretch both sides!

of motion, which will prevent injuries from all aspects of daily life. Muscles can also benefit from being stretched within the limits of their natural boundaries. Tendons shrink if not regularly put to the test, which can lead to overall stiffness and rigidity. You may notice this feeling when you wake up in the morning. A little stiffness here, a little soreness there. I often wake up from a wonderful night's sleep and stand beside my bed doing stretches while I watch *Robin & Company* on CNN. Somehow I feel better having given my body that extra stretch time right off the bat.

Try to do six 5-minute stretch sessions each week to attain ultimate flexibility. You can do these exercises any time. They are not tiring or particularly difficult. And remember, stretching needs to be maintained

– you can take one step forward by stretching and two steps back by missing a session.

In general, pre-workout stretching should be dynamic (stretches in which you rhythmically move and extend your natural reach – for example, swinging your arms). Post-workout stretches should be static (stretches in which you stay fairly motionless except to reach slightly further – for example, touching your toes) since muscles are already warm and are more elastic.

On pages 38 and 39 are just a few examples of static stretches. However, you should stretch out every muscle you exercise after your workout.

TIP

I simply keep a pair of my favorite dress pants and jeans handy to measure where I'm at!

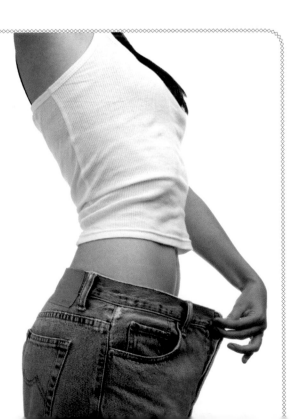

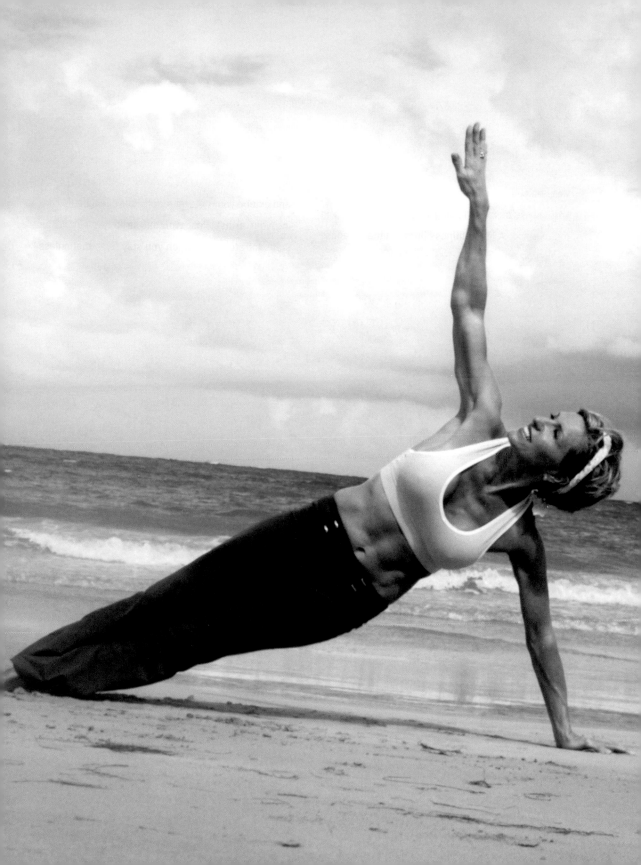

STRETCHES

Swan Lift

This stretch is not as popular as it used to be, but it's great for stretching the quadriceps, abdomen, front delts and chest, all at once. It also works to strengthen the extensors of the lower back and the glutes. Whew! Lie on your stomach, bend your legs, reach back and grab hold of your ankles. Pull your ankles and lift your head off the floor at the same time.

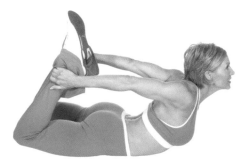

Glute Stretch

This great glute stretch, called "thread the needle," is commonly used in yoga. Lie on your back with your knees bent and feet on the floor. Rest your right ankle just above your left knee. Clasp your hands behind your left knee and gently pull it towards you. You should feel a stretch in your right glute. Repeat on other side.

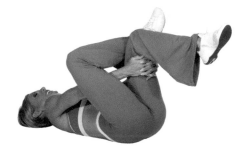

Hamstrings Stretch

The hamstrings stretch will target the back of your thigh. Sit on the floor. Extend your left leg, with toes pointing to the ceiling. Place the sole of your right foot against the inside of your left leg. Reach toward your left foot, trying to touch your knee with your nose. Repeat on the other side.

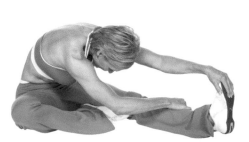

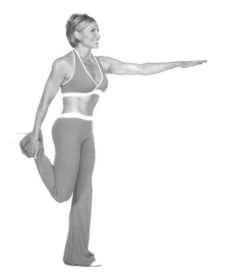

Quadriceps Stretch

The quadriceps stretch will stretch the front of your thigh. Stand up and place one hand against the wall. Reach behind with your other hand, grab your ankle and pull your foot toward your backside. Make sure your hips and pelvis are in line.

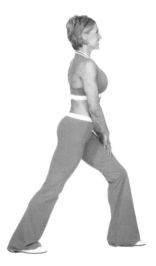

Calf Stretch

The calf stretch will target the back of your lower leg. Standing, step back with your right foot. Keeping your leg straight, try to push your heel to the floor. Repeat with your left foot.

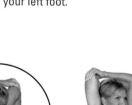

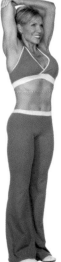

Triceps Stretch

You may sit or stand for the exercise. Lift one arm above your head and bend your elbow. Use the opposite hand to pull your elbow toward your head until you feel a stretch along the back of your arm. Make sure to stretch the other triceps!

Easy Does It

Whenever you perform stretching exercises it is important not to bounce yourself into the stretched position – this is called ballistic stretching, and it can be harmful. The idea is to stretch out, gradually making demands on your joints, ligaments, and muscles, but not subjecting them to traumatic jolts by bouncing. Regular stretching can actually help prevent injuries because you strengthen the vulnerable areas (injuries in weight training commonly occur as a result of overextension), but do not expect to get overnight results. Research has shown that significant results do not make themselves evident for at least three to six weeks after commencement of a stretching program. So you see why you have to commit to stretching right from the start.

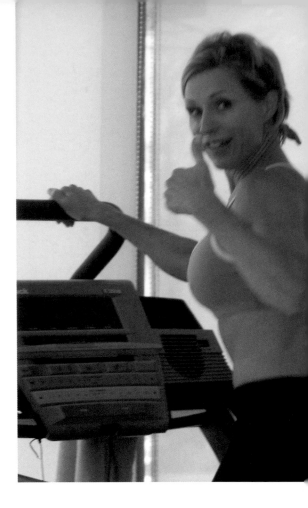

Stretching before training is a good idea and fits in well with rope jumping and other cardiovascular exercise, but do not neglect the importance of stretching after your workout. Even a little stretching is better than none, so make an effort. This promotes even more flexibility because a warm muscle responds better to the stretching effect; it also serves to help slowly cool down the body, something physiologists believe is just as important as warming up.

Pre-Exercise Warm-up

As well as stretching and warming up, you should complete warm-up sets for each exercise you do. This simply means that the first set of each exercise

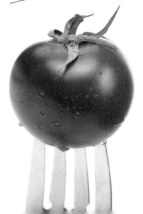

TIP

To help training results stick, Eat Clean every day!

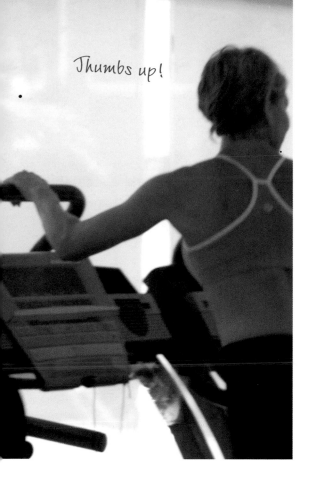

Thumbs up!

using maximum-intensity training. My first set may not be terribly impressive but it certainly makes me focus on the iron in front of me. The next set is better but the third is usually the money set. I get stronger as the muscles warm up and become fully engaged in the effort at hand. I feel really good right then and you will find this happening to you too.

Better Performance

If you take the time to stretch and warm up properly before and after a workout, your body will perform better and recover from strenuous exercise more effectively. Many of you like to set the tone for training by doing a 5-minute cardio warmup before stretching a single muscle or touching a weight. This is a wonderful way to wake up your body and get your active juices flowing. I like to skip or do plyometric jumps before a workout. That means I am good and warm by the time I reach for my first dumbell.

should be done with about half the regular weight and twice as many reps. I love the first set because it gets me in the groove of what I am about to do. It helps me transition from my previous activity. The first light-and-loose set will help prevent the muscle injury that could occur if you immediately start with a heavy set of exercise.

Older people may find that more than one warm-up set is needed, especially on heavy exercises such as squats, deadlifts and bench presses. If you are troubled by weak knees you should warm up your legs with several sets of each leg exercise before

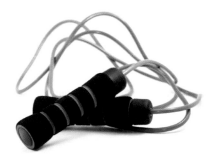

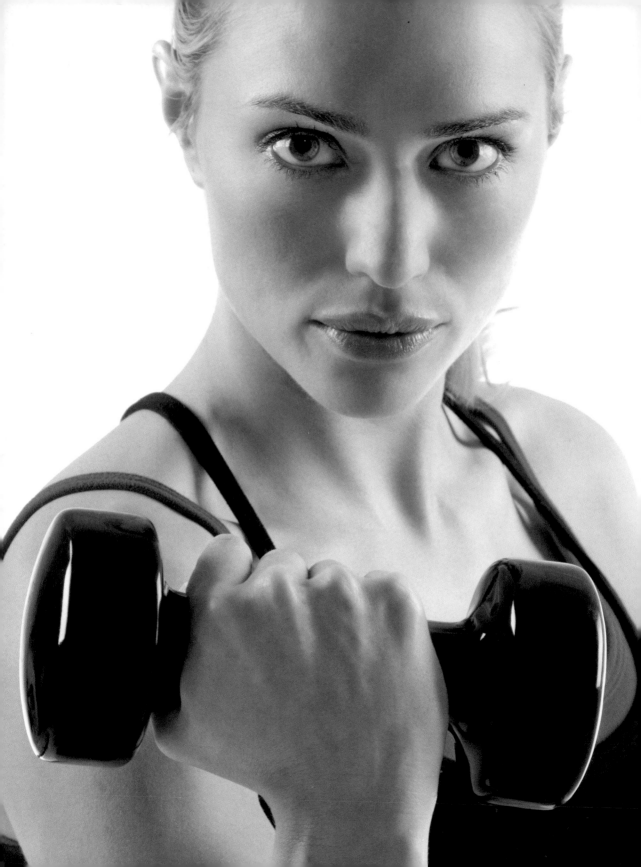

2

"Once you get the hang of it, resistance training is no more difficult or intimidating than riding a bike or jumping on your treadmill."

SETS AND REPS
THE ESSENCE OF TRAINING

I n bodybuilding there are a thousand and one ways to train, but training without any type of plan is not one of them. If you are determined to be successful you must plan for it. Your first steps here will plot the course of your physique-renovation journey.

Sets and reps are the heart and soul of resistance exercise. They are the framework of your routine. When you consider that the possible combinations of sets, reps and exercises are infinite – well, it can all seem very complicated. How many exercises should you do? How many sets and reps? You could do just three exercises, or one hundred. The possible number of sets for each exercise may range from one to twenty. Reps can run the gamut from one to several hundred. Like snowflakes, no two routines are identical. Even training partners performing the same program often do different numbers of sets and reps. You will even do varying numbers of sets and reps on different days, depending on how strong you feel.

Perfect Routine?

People want to find the perfect routine for themselves. They also love learning the routines of the champs, in the hope that duplicating them will create a similar type of prize-winning physique.

It's worth saying here and now, to give you peace of mind: Following Maggie Diubaldo's routine will not give you a body like Maggie's. Your routines may be

"Keep in mind that your routine evolves and continually changes. Changes, small and large, are a very real part of each workout."

the same but their effect is governed by physiological characteristics, not to mention exercise style, genetic aptitude and nutrition habits. I encourage you to train for your own reasons and to achieve your ultimate body – not someone else's. You will get nothing but frustration and disappointment from the other approach. Remember, this is about you and you only!

Keep in mind that your routine evolves and continually changes. Changes, small and large, are a very real part of each workout. Do not make the common mistake of thinking that there exists a magic routine that will transform you into an instant Ms. Universe. Even the pros don't have the ideal workout – they chop and change continually.

A Good Base

But you must start somewhere! Develop a good routine as a base from which to work. The important point is that any new routine should under-stress the body rather than overstress it. This will keep injuries to a minimum. As you become more experienced you can train harder.

Here are some basic truths to keep in mind as you create your routine. Sets of low reps (1 to 6) contribute greatly to increased strength. Medium reps (7 to 12) build muscle size. High reps (13 to 200) will build mitochondrial size and overall conditioning. Please keep in mind that these reps should be relatively difficult. I can't tell you how many times I've seen women do 12 reps of an exercise with a weight so light they could have done 100 reps. That is missing the point entirely! When you do 12 reps, a 13th rep should be almost impossible. Another common misconception is that women think medium reps build, therefore high reps tone. Baloney! High reps will not define muscles. This is accomplished by incorporating Clean Eating in conjunction with consistent training.

Here are some ideas of how many sets and reps to perform depending on your experience. Remember this is a guideline only. Expect to play with your numbers a lot, and bear in mind that there is no magic formula. Your routine, whether you are a beginner, intermediate, or advanced trainer, is an evolving structure. It should change frequently to accommodate the advances made by your body.

BEGINNER

Beginners should start with light, easy weights and perform only one set of 8 to 12 repetitions per exercise. Never strain or take on more than you can comfortably handle. After two weeks you can graduate to 2 sets of 8 to 12 reps. Continue with this for a month or two.

INTERMEDIATE

After two months of training, your body has been sufficiently immersed in regular workouts for you to increase the number of sets and weight even more. At this stage 3 or 4 sets per exercise is about average. Keep the reps between 8 and 12.

ADVANCED

Here's where we get rid of the rules. Advanced women generally have to subject their muscles to more work than intermediates do, but not indefinitely. More sets and reps are not necessarily better. You may find that training as you did at the intermediate level is still beneficial, with the added twist of increasing the intensity of each set.

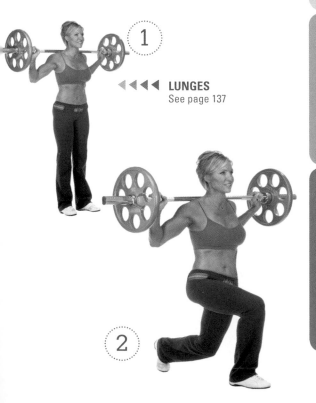

◀◀◀◀ **LUNGES**
See page 137

On the other hand, you may go up to 5 or 6 sets per exercise. Advanced trainers have several alternative routes to take (and rules to break if they are so inclined). You could keep to 3 sets per exercise but increase the number of exercises. Or you could vary the number of sets per exercise in order to work on an underdeveloped area (add more sets) or go easy on a well-developed area (do fewer sets).

You will likely want to change your repetition range depending on which muscle group you are exercising. As an advanced trainer you may discover that your thighs will respond best to a system of 10 to 15 reps. Your calves, abdominals and forearms may require 15 to 20 reps per set, while your upper body muscles may thrive best on 8 to 12 reps.

These suggestions are not meant to be law, but are indicative of what women have generally found to be the most useful. Until you find out more about your own body, follow those who know! I am still working on my ideal routine, since I have discovered that the older I get the more things change. I play around with exercise until I feel good about the results I am getting. And hey, I am exercising! That's the point, isn't it?

Training Style and Pace

Training style helps prevent injury if you follow good form. Good form can also greatly benefit your development. What is good form? It is the lifting of a weight from start to finish in a smooth manner, using only

THREE CHEATING MOVEMENTS YOU SHOULD NEVER DO

TO ENSURE SAFETY:

1 When performing the preacher curl, never "drop" the weight as the arm straightens in the low position. This can cause catastrophic tendon or biceps injury. Lower the weight under complete (slow) control for every repetition.

2 During the bench press, never bounce the bar on your breastbone (sternum) to help the weight upward. You can badly bruise or even crack your rib cage.

3 When squatting, never bounce your upper legs against your lower legs in the low part of the exercise. This is just too hard on the knees and will eventually cause injury.

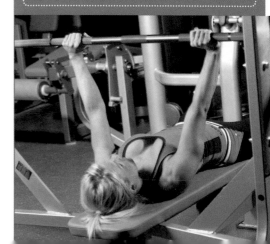

the muscles directly involved in the lift. You cannot bend your knees and throw up a weight. You cannot bounce the bar on your body to give it momentum.

For example, a strict curl starts with the bar held in front of the thighs, with straight, locked arms and legs. The bar is then curled (raised) by moving only the forearms. The upper arm is held vertically against the side. The trunk (upper body) remains vertical throughout. This strict form forces the biceps to do the majority of the work rather than other muscles that might like to get involved if you are not careful.

Contrast a strict curl with a cheat curl. When you perform a cheat curl (loose style) you start with your arms slightly bent, torso leaning forward, knees bent. As you begin the curl you straighten, your knees, lean your torso forward, and rock your torso back to aid in the curling action.

As a beginner, you should perform all your exercises in very strict style. Later, as you learn how your body reacts to various exercises, you may find it advantageous to cheat during the last few reps on some exercises. This is once you find that you just cannot perform any more strict repetitions but still want to push out a few more.

Strict or Cheat?

The golden rule about exercise performance is simply that you should use the exercise style that will best fully stimulate your muscles. This means that, for the most part, your exercises should be

> **"Never forget that healthy muscles adapt very quickly to strict exercise."**

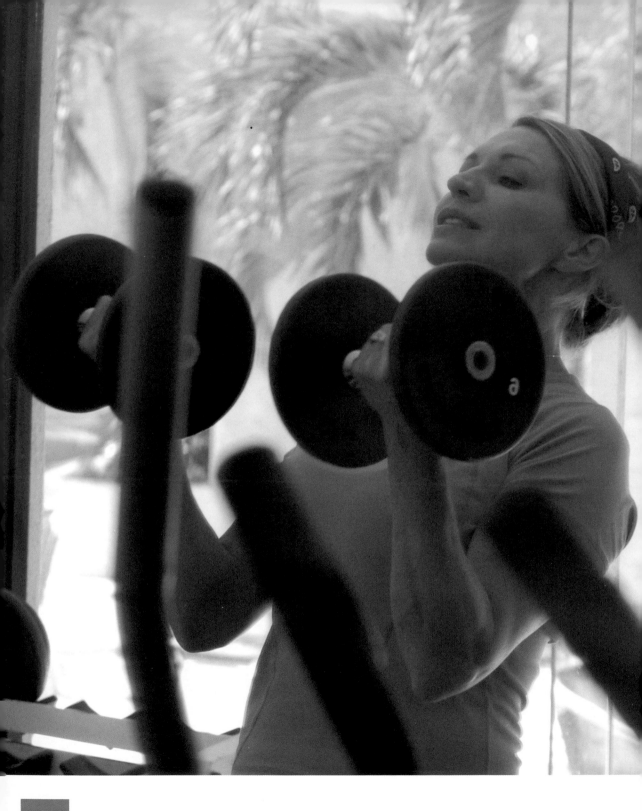

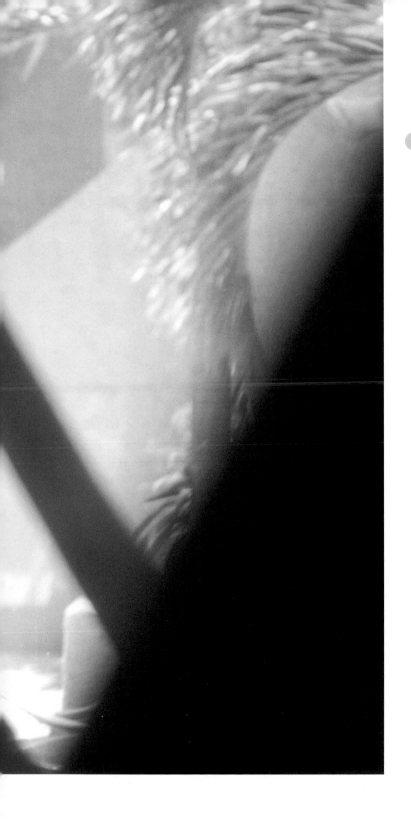

TIP

I take pride in doing my best work at all times, especially in the gym.

performed strictly, using a full range of motion and exercising in a rhythmic and smooth fashion. At the same time there is merit in occasionally using loose form in some exercises. We call this controlled creative cheating.

Let's say you are in the middle of a set of curls. You have done 5 very strict reps and cannot do another one. You could put the weight down (and not get the full benefit of 8 to 12 reps) or you could loosen up your style and continue. Even though in cheating the curl upwards you take much of the effect away from the biceps, you can still stress the muscle maximally as you lower the weight slowly (known as the negative effect). In fact sometimes I get a beautiful sweet pain from doing negatives – the final deliberately slow lowering of the barbell.

Never forget that healthy muscles adapt very quickly to strict exercise. You do need to change training style, sets, reps, and exercises fairly frequently. Strict, high-intensity, quality training, however, should form the basis of your workout. Controlled cheating can be used on occasion when you will benefit. Moderation is the key here. If you cheat in every exercise, you will get nowhere fast.

Workout Pace

Training pace is the rate at which you progress through your routine. There are more variations than you may think. First, how quickly should you execute your repetitions? There is a great deal of heated argument over this question, because successful trainers seem to find that both quick reps and slow reps work well.

The beginner should not try to exercise quickly. The "groove" (the path the weight travels in each exercise) must be established before you can do speed reps. If you are using really heavy weights for low reps, don't work at a fast pace. As time goes on and you learn how to *feel* your exercise as you lift the weight, you can work at a faster rate to complete your workout sooner, but this requires intimate knowledge of what your body is capable of handling.

The ideal rest period between sets is 30 to 90 seconds.

Rest Between Sets

It is important to rest between your sets and exercises. You should start the next set when your breathing returns to normal. Unfortunately some trainers have interpreted this as resting for up to 10 minutes between each set! If I did that I would never get my workouts done, nor would I get any work done. I don't have that kind of time and I'm pretty sure you don't either. I get down to business when I am in the gym because I know I have only so much time and I have to make it count.

The less you rest between each group of repetitions, the more stress you place on your muscles, but more is not always better. If you train too rapidly, you will outrun your muscular system. In other words, you will be benefiting your heart and lungs at the expense of your muscles. The oxygen debt, deep breathing and accompanying discomfort will hold you back from doing justice to the muscles being trained.

On the other hand, training slowly with very long rests between sets will cause your energy level to drop. You could even find yourself yawning. I've seen that plenty of times in the big meat-monster gyms. The ideal rest period between sets is 30 to 90 seconds. You will need to rest a little more between heavy combination exercises for large muscle groups, such as squats, bench presses, rows, and dead lifts, and I am excited to tell you that you may rest up to a full five minutes between working out different body parts. For example, after working your thighs with various exercises, resting briefly between each, you may subsequently take a break of five minutes or so before moving on to, say, back training. The same goes for every body part – arms, shoulders, chest,

TIP

Strive only to be the best you possible! It is exciting to discover what that is.

abs. Take a breather before moving on to the next area. This allows the blood (also known as the pump) to stay in the region for a while until you move on to another section. What is the point of this? The blood feeds the muscle with nutrients needed to repair them. The break also refreshes! When you progress to another area of the body, go back to resting 30 to 90 seconds between sets.

Finding the right number of sets and reps is an ever-changing process. However, as you perform your routines your body will let you know when the time is right for a change. You may have to experiment by adding reps or sets here and there and discovering "Hey, I can do that! Next time I'll do 15 calf raises instead of 12."

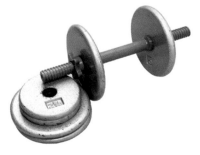

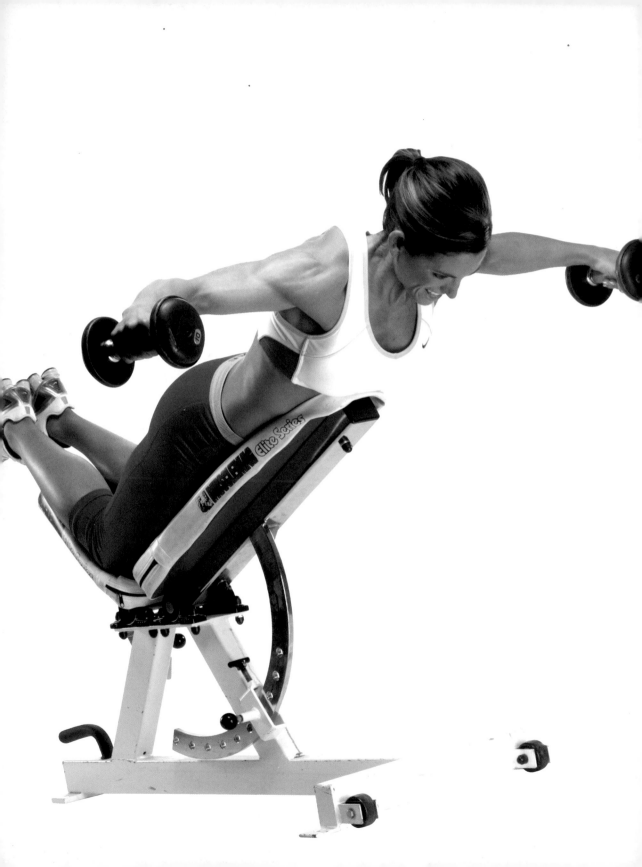

3

"I invite you to attend the party of your own life. Put on your best face. Eat Clean until you gleam and shine. Be there! Dance like no one is watching and do it every day."

PSYCHO POWER
THE MAGIC OF THE MIND

According to exercise expert Robert Kennedy: "The mind is one of the most awesome and powerful forces on earth. Properly utilized, your mind can help you build one of the greatest bodies in the world." I believe that. What's more, I subscribe to it with all I do. Just being on this side of the dirt reminds me of the power and potential of the human mind.

The brain controls everything we do and we can program it with goals, orders, even enthusiasm. Without the correct positive attitude you will not reach your dreams.

Regardless of their position in life, all successful people practice the art of positive thinking. If you do not *believe* you can do something, then you never will. Start now by telling yourself that you are going

> **❝ The mind is one of the most awesome and powerful forces on earth. Properly utilized, your mind can help you build one of the greatest bodies in the world. ❞**

There is no doubt that the mind can control the body's physical reactions to outside stimuli. A tuned mind can render a body impervious to heat, as evidenced by people who can walk on red-hot coals and not feel pain. It can stimulate the release of adrenaline from visualization of fear. As a result of that burst of adrenalin, a person can lift a car off someone pinned underneath, or perform other superhuman feats. In Africa, doctors of traditional medicine (who are totally revered) can cure or curse believers with nothing more than a chanted spell.

Program Your Mind

You can use your mind in your quest for physical perfection. First you must prepare yourself to be who you want to be. Your mind is your own personal computer and only you can program it for success.

to develop a great-looking body with robust health and that you will let nothing stop you. Next you must believe in yourself! Practice saying, "I can do it!" Soon enough you will truly believe you can!

"Most people are their own worst enemies," says fitness expert Kim Lyons. "They stand in the way of their own progress. The standard cop-out is: 'I could never succeed at that, so I won't even try.'" You must immerse yourself in positive thoughts when you train your body. Success is yours for the taking, but it won't come about from a sloppy attitude. A workout is serious. You can't take time off between sets to read a book or watch television. Don't get in the habit of talking and joking. Don't even feel obligated to respond to anyone. Politely tell them not to talk to you while you are training, and they will get the message. My favorite trick to avoid these awkward

TIP

Don't let age stop you from being your best. Remember I didn't start weight training until the age of 40!

moments is to put the earbuds from my iPod in my ears (even if I am not listening to music). I have a hard time saying no and the iPod tells folks I can't hear them.

Before every set, tell yourself how many reps you will accomplish with a given weight. This doesn't mean you go all out for every set, but you must program your mind and tune in your concentration for every set. The positive practice of concentrating on your goals builds good neuromuscular efficiency, strong nerve pathways, and your mind-to-muscle relationship improves, all of which adds to your performance level and, ultimately, superior results.

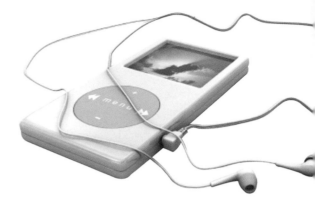

The Enthusiasm Factor

Many women assume that if they train with enough enthusiasm, motivation and intensity, their gains and progress will never cease. This is one of the most misguided ideas in training today.

Too much intensity cuts short your progress faster than anything else. After only a few workouts your body presses the alarm button and nervous exhaustion sets in. The same goes for workouts that are too long in duration, or training frequency that does not allow for sufficient rest. These practices cause severe overtraining, which inevitably results in frustration, disillusionment and possible injury. Many women make no improvement despite super-hard efforts. A return of zero from 100 percent commitment is heartbreaking, but it happens all the time.

Progress comes from intense training, but this training must be tailored to your condition. Never let your emotions carry you through a workout – trying for records, doubling your efforts, extending your workout time. Unless these advances are made with small progressive steps you will be doomed to early failure. It is easy for over-enthusiasm to take the place of common sense. However, you must not allow yourself to become too relaxed, either. Progress comes from intelligent hard training, using prudence and caution.

Listen to Your Body

Tolerance to exercise varies: too much for one woman can be totally inadequate for another. This brings us to the topic of body feedback. The more you learn about your reaction to exercise, the better you will tailor your workouts to your individual needs. If you feel drained when you are due for your next workout, you are likely overtraining. Cut back. Exercise with more moderation and make sure your diet is free of junk food.

Motivation

The attainment of lean muscle, strength, beauty and health is the right of every woman. It is an honest endeavor. Some women have the need to build a superb body deep within their souls. They are filled with motivation. At some point, however, this need may desert them – after having kids, or as they get busy with other activities. They still want that dynamite body, but the all-encompassing need is not there. They may ask themselves if the reward is worth the effort.

If you are going through this you need to summon the power of the mind. Remind yourself of your original goals. Pull out that photo of a younger, leaner, happier you. Then remember the promise you made to yourself. With enough mental effort, you can remake your body into anything your genetic endowment permits. It's a question of mind over matter! Read

The more you learn about your reaction **to exercise, the better you** will tailor your **workouts to your** individual needs.

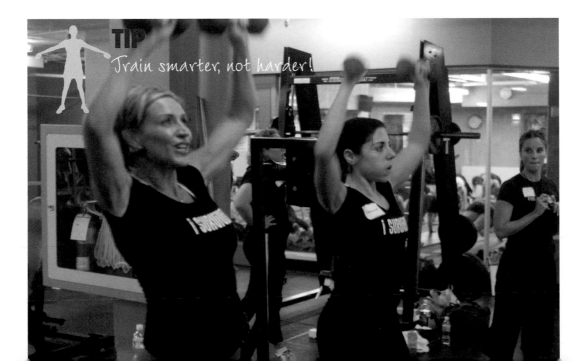

TIP
Train smarter, not harder!

books and magazines on training. Study the pictures of top fit women you admire. Don't just flick through the pages – picture yourself *on* the pages. Imagine the glory of fame. Fire up your ambitions! Fuel your desire to the hilt! You don't have to tell the world. It can be our little secret.

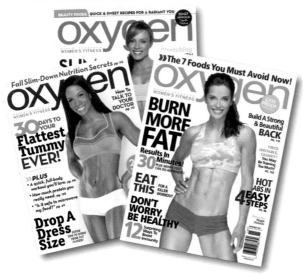

▶▶▶ **NEVER MISS AN ISSUE OF *OXYGEN* MAGAZINE.**

If your ambition is simply to rebuild your body to a shape you are happy with, that is enough. You may be a mother whose children deserve the healthiest, happiest mom possible. Training made me a better mom. I was bitter and angry at the world. I was unhappy. I missed my former athletic self who had disappeared behind a pile of diapers and laundry. At a little over 200 pounds I never imagined I could lose enough weight to recreate a healthier me. I was sure I was destined to lard for the rest of my life. It was

only when I discarded self-destructive habits and embraced new ones like Clean Eating and weight training that I believed another me was even possible. It *was* possible, and I ask you now to believe in yourself for a minute and dare to hope that your life can be the one you have dreamed of deep inside your soul.

Try Something New

A lack of inspiration can be overcome in many ways. Try training in a different setting – at a friend's house or a new gym. Some women find it inspirational to train with a male workout partner. "It stirs up the hormones," says one top woman champ. "I'm not going to give up on a set until it's completed if I know some guy is counting the reps for me." Consider training with a group of supportive women. They have a way of keeping you honest, and slacking off won't be tolerated.

Keep up to date on women's fitness. Never miss an issue of *Oxygen* magazine. The points of view will keep you abreast of the latest trends and the photographs will inspire you to unbelievable achievement. I love to share my stories of training and nutrition in "Raise the Bar," a column I was supposed to write for women in their 40s but that draws readers of both sexes, aged 8 to 88. No kidding!

Check out the Competition

When I accepted my first challenge to enter a bodybuilding competition I watched loads of exercise and competition videotapes. Studying other women's physiques and exercise styles helped me determine what I wanted for my own physique. In the beginning I did not know how my own body would look at its best. In the end I discovered I wanted broad shoulders, popping delts, beautiful wide lats tapering into a narrow waist, and flowing quads. I had to go to shows to figure that out.

TIP

I love the idea of a contest but I often tell those interested in competing to do it for the journey, not necessarily to win.

You may want to do so as well. There are bound to be several NPC (National Physique Committee) contests in your area for amateur fitness and figure women. Professional shows are well worth visiting, even if it means traveling some distance to attend. You will never forget the excitement of a Ms. Olympia fitness contest. Training to lose fat and muscle up is your hobby. You are choosing to live this life. Decide now to be a part of it in every way.

When you really believe in yourself, when you're inspired and completely determined to achieve your goal, your mind releases the amount of energy you need to give it your best shot. And you can't ask for anything more than that!

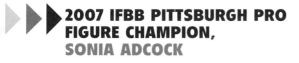

2007 IFBB PITTSBURGH PRO FIGURE CHAMPION, SONIA ADCOCK

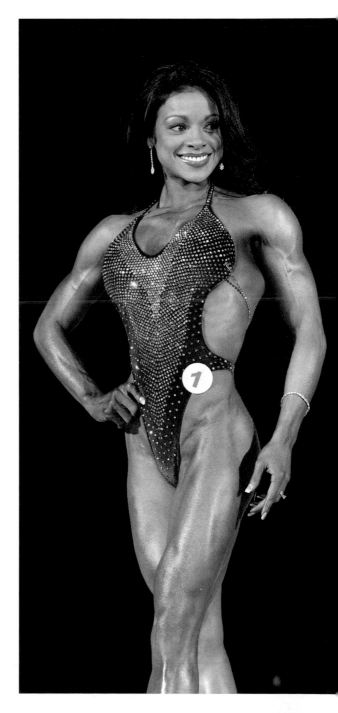

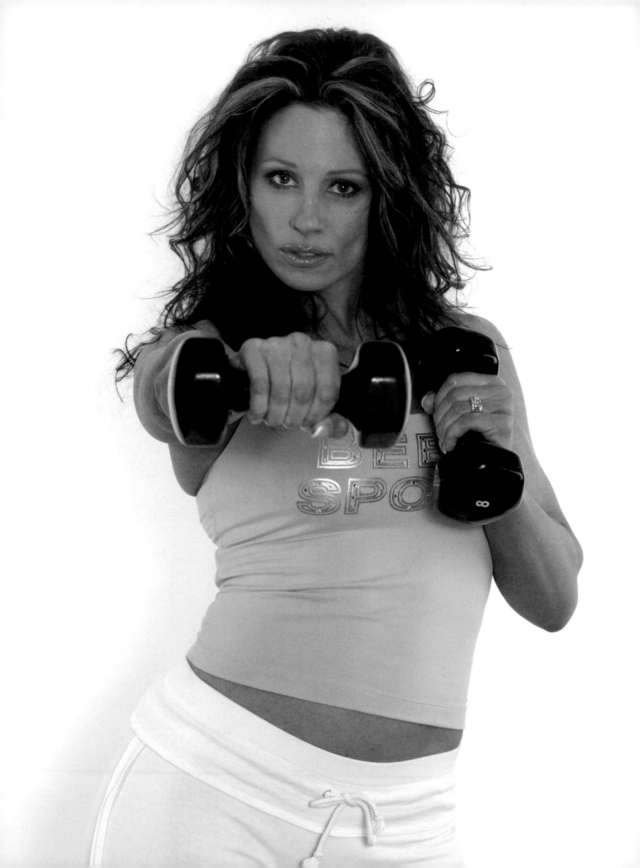

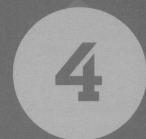

4

"Life is pretty exhausting and 'stuff' just keeps coming. Guess what? You can turn it off for a bit and take your chunk of the day to look after you. No excuses!"

TOUGHING IT OUT
REGULAR WORKOUTS ARE A MUST

Perseverance is your key to success in fitness. Results come at varying speeds, but they will not come at all if you do not persist with regular workouts.

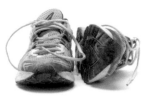

Changes sometimes come so slowly, especially at the beginning, you will be sorely tempted to quit. Early on in my training I expected instant perfection. Because they were my stubborn areas, I trained my legs and buttocks five days a week. I did squats, uphill sprints, leg extensions … I was so discouraged at the slow progress that I hid my legs under sweat pants. It wasn't till I met publisher Robert Kennedy that I realized less could be more. Once I began training my legs and glutes just twice a week I soon saw steady progress.

Set Your Goals

The first thing to put into practice is goal setting. Do not set impossible goals, because failing to reach them can undermine anyone's self-esteem. Stay within the boundaries of attainable results. It's far better to understate a goal and achieve it quickly than to set an impossible task and doom yourself to failure.

Keep the list in a highly visible area (on your fridge or in the bathroom). A goal is a commitment to stay on course. Allocate yourself a time by which each goal must be met. By committing yourself to bench press 20 pounds more in six weeks, for example, you are increasing the urgency of the promise.

Have pictures taken of yourself every few months. They will serve to remind you of how far you have come and where you are going. With the help of regular picture taking you will be fully aware of your condition – and the improvements you've been making!

SET YOUR GOALS IN TWO PARTS
(SEE GOAL SHEETS ON PAGE 216)

1 WRITE DOWN YOUR LONG-TERM GOAL
(ie. getting a 28-inch waist, competing in a figure contest, wearing size-6 jeans)

_____

2 WRITE DOWN YOUR INTERIM GOALS
(ie. adding 20 pounds to your bench press in six weeks, going to the gym consistently for one month, decreasing your body-fat percentage by three percent by the end of the winter)

Keep a Record

You should also keep a training log. Record your exercises, sets, reps and weights for every workout. I can review eight years of my training with a flick of the pages! That's pretty handy information. A training log should be used to keep you informed about your workouts – what worked, what didn't – and to allow you to see your progress. You should cycle your training for utmost benefit, planning your workouts to gradually increase intensity as you aim for a particular peak. After you reach that peak you can taper off, or "down cycle" your training for a while.

A training log should record everything – not just your sets, reps, and poundages, but how the workout felt. Were you tired, overheated, drained, or did the sets come easily? I make a note if something happened that may affect my training performance. Was I up late the night before? Had I been traveling? Did I eat something different that morning?

When you achieve a new record in a workout, put a star beside the appropriate set. These stars will indicate your progress. Record your measurements and weight every month or two, but don't make the miserable mistake of weighing and measuring yourself every day, or even every week. Record diet changes, supplements, and any injuries. State whether you cheated during an exercise. A training journal is a useful tool. Most of the better trainers keep a record to maximize their progress. You can find journal

pages to photocopy on page 214. *The Eat-Clean Diet Workout Journal* can be found in most online and retail bookstores.

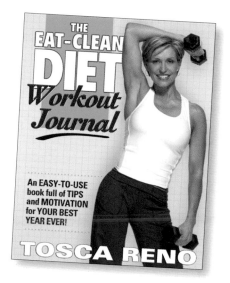

Music for Energy

Are your workouts dragging? Listening to music will likely help. Scientific evidence shows that the right music will help you breeze through a workout that might otherwise be boring. Certainly cardio is easier when performed to music. I can't imagine running HIITs without my iPod – I lose myself in the music and before I know it several miles have flown by.

Finally, if you come up with a problem that you cannot find an answer to, ask others for advice. Attend seminars and camps, read avidly and gather as much knowledge as you can about fitness. When you are totally immersed in the iron game, you will stick to it with no problem. Remember, once you train with weights you have joined a powerful group of women called "Sisters in Iron."

Home or Gym Training?

Most serious fitness women train at commercial gyms. However, at least a portion of their training time in the beginning was spent at home, in the garage or basement, often with only the bare necessities of a bench and a set of dumbells. Both locations, home and gym, have advantages. Don't overlook one for the other.

Home training is convenient. You can do your workout whenever the urge hits. You have the advantage of total privacy if you feel uncomfortable exercising in front of others. Yet you have to be totally dedicated if you train at home, especially if you have kids. There is always something calling you! Besides, it's so easy to relax, turn on the TV and presto! You become too lazy to get started. Missed workouts become commonplace and before you know it your progress has gone into reverse. We also tend not to work out as hard at home.

A commercial gym, on the other hand, has a competitive atmosphere. You invariably train with more intensity where other people are exercising. There may be times you really can't make it, but in general taking your workouts to a good gym is the faster way to reach your goal. One factor against the commercial-training setup is the possibility of overcrowding. Monday nights are notorious for this, because many members take weekends off from their training and are then anxious to get back in.

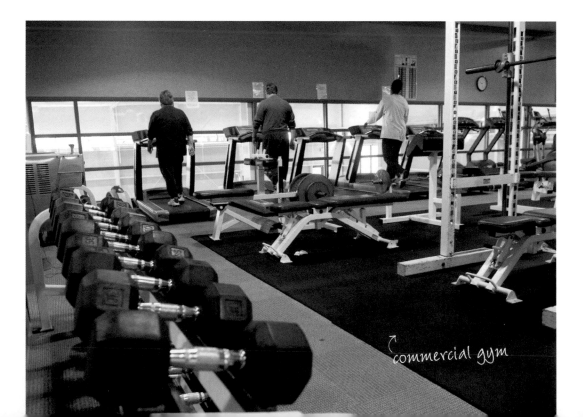

commercial gym

Monday nights are worst for cardio hogs — people who take more than their fair share of time on the cardio equipment, leaving you frustrated.

If you are shy you may like the refuge of training at home, but remember that there are always people in worse shape than you. Besides, no one will be looking at you. Gym-goers are normally far too busy catching sight of themselves in the mirrors to worry about anyone else!

More Reasons to Join

For the most part, temperature will be balanced in a commercial gym (you may not have air conditioning at home). Then there's the variety of equipment. Although barbells and dumbells can certainly be effective on their own, a variety of apparatus, including pulleys, leg machines, etc., can be a valuable contribution to the ultimate success of your physique renovation. Some gyms also have the added bonus of a pool. The pool is one of my favorite places to get a wicked cardio session.

> The luxury of fixed dumbells, set out in rows, graduating in 5-pound increments, is hard to beat.

A gym will have a greater variety of fixed dumbells and barbells. This will save you the somewhat tedious job of changing plates every time you want to alter poundages. The luxury of fixed dumbells, set

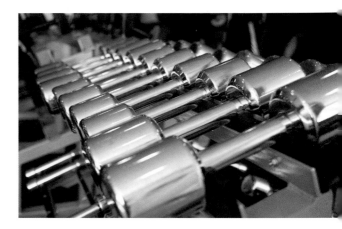

out in rows, graduating in 5-pound increments, is hard to beat.

What to Look For

Before joining a gym, find out exactly what you get for your money. You may discover that the basic annual fee doesn't entitle you to use all the facilities. Also, consider the distance to the gym. Would winter weather prove a problem? Would travel to and from the gym take too much time and prevent you from getting there?

Does your gym membership include personal instruction? This is very important to some people, but others may resent an instructor telling them what to do. Some establishments insist that you exercise in the style they dictate. If you are an experienced trainer, this may rub you the wrong way. Check out the gym's policy before joining.

How do you know whether you are considering a good or a bad gym? If there are a lot of electrical de-

TIP

Use your gym as a source of information and motivation. Good gyms often bring in special guests from the fitness industry who can help you fine-tune your physique goals. Your gym might also post special events and fitness contests — something you may want to consider entering!

vices such as vibrator belts and roller machines and the salesman insists these will help you lose pounds, forget it. The main tools for body shaping are barbells, dumbells, cardio areas, benches, pulleys, and sturdy exercise stations.

A thick pile carpet, soft music, chrome apparatus and air conditioning are not necessities for a good gym, but if atmosphere is important to you then pay attention. If you feel uncomfortable in a gym then you probably won't go, no matter how adequate the equipment. Look for simple, strong apparatus and an enthusiastic group of people training. Note I did not say young people. People of all ages should be enjoying the facility.

If everyone on the gym floor is talking, chances are you will be doing the same. Look for a busy training area that will inspire you to train hard and make progress. The clanging of weights on the gym floor is the right music – not Frank Sinatra singing "My Way" while the gym members sit around the juice bar gossiping or reading *People* magazine.

Check the gym's hours. Ideally, a gym should be open at least six (and preferably seven) days a week. I am not suggesting you train daily, but it's nice to know that if you have to miss a workout, you can always return the next day.

It's Your Money

Most gyms today are honorable and reliable. In the past, this was not always the case. But the prime concern of any commercial gym is the same

Look for a busy training area that will inspire you to train hard and make progress.

as ever: to make money. You must ask yourself: "Do they give value for my money?"

If a pushy salesperson counters your negative reply with a question (this is a sales tactic), you are quite within your rights to say politely: "Look, I don't have to explain or justify myself in any way. I have told you I will think about it, and if I decide to join I will let you know."

Gym fees vary greatly. Shop around and compare. If you decide to set up a gym at home, then buy equipment that is made by a well-known and respected company. Try it out and make sure it feels comfortable and suits your needs. Do not buy what you are unlikely to use. Once you have made the decision to join a gym or set up your own home-training apparatus, remember that your persistence is the key to your success.

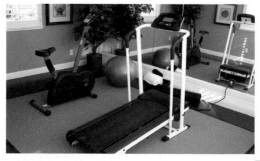

home gym

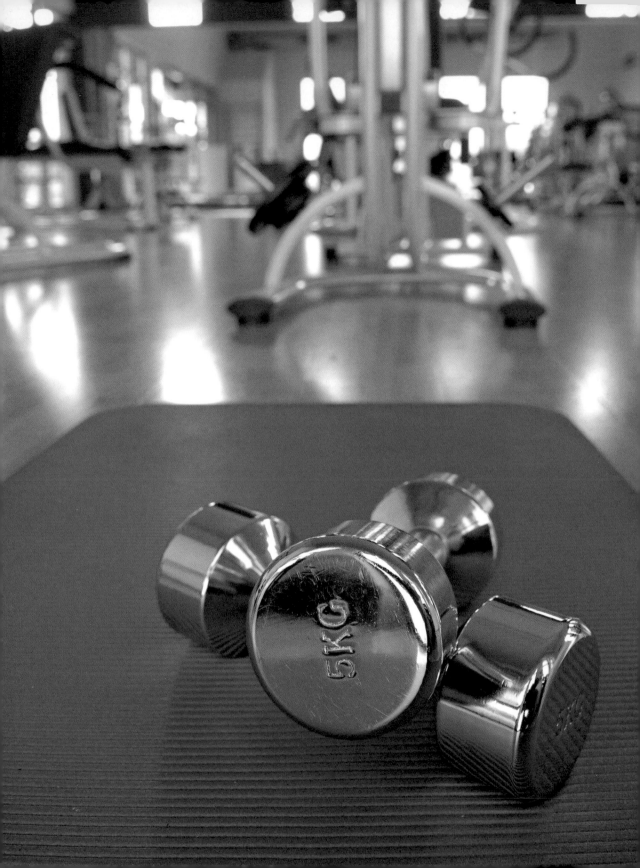

5

"The connection I have made with weights and resistance training equipment has made me one of the millions of 'Sisters in Iron' worldwide. When I began, every rep I performed and each set I completed helped me rebuild my self-esteem. Training with weights literally saved my life."

GADGETS GALORE
BODYBUILDING TOOLS

Name any sport, hobby, or pastime and you will find a bounty of accessory items. Fitness workouts are no different. I am often asked what the minimum requirements are for a woman to start weight training. The absolute necessities are: a barbell set, several pairs of dumbells and an exercise bench (preferably one that adjusts easily to an incline). A pair of squat stands are a bonus if you have room. The barbell set should contain at least 110 pounds of weights. You should have sets of 5-pound, 10-pound, 15-pound, and 20-pound dumbells. Later you may want to add sets of 25s and 30s. That's it. You're in business.

Of course, as you get into training you will acquire additional accessories. Items such as gloves, elbow and knee braces and lifting straps may not have direct bearing on your training progress, but they can make your workouts more pleasurable.

I advise you not to skimp on the necessities, but buy accessories only as you can afford them. You need a weight set and a bench and preferably squat racks. They are an investment rather than an expense.

TRAINING AIDS

Weight-Training Belts

Once you start training with heavier weights, a good-quality weight belt is invaluable. All serious trainers wear a belt, especially for exercises such as dead lifts, rows and squats. Some women wear a belt throughout their entire workout, but you can just use it for certain basic exercises if you wish.

Belts, usually leather, are available in 4-inch (10-cm) and 6-inch (15-cm) widths (occasionally larger). A woman really shouldn't need anything wider than a 4-inch belt. A weight belt helps protect the lower back by giving additional support. It also increases your confidence when lifting heavier poundages, and contributes in a positive way to increasing strength.

MINIMUM EQUIPMENT REQUIREMENTS

- ⋯⟩ **BARBELL SET**
- ⋯⟩ **SEVERAL PAIRS OF DUMBELLS**
- ⋯⟩ **EXERCISE BENCH** *(PREFERABLY AN ADJUSTABLE INCLINE BENCH)*

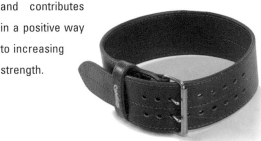

I like to wear a weight belt when doing squats. That is the only time I wear one during my training.

Gloves

The first person to regularly wear training gloves was bodybuilder Serge Nubret, of France. The idea didn't catch on quickly but nowadays most trainers wear them. These special half-finger gloves form a barrier between the sweat of your hands and the slippery surface of the bar. They also help prevent calluses. I am never without gloves unless I'm training my legs.

I rarely train with bare hands — mostly because I'm too lazy to remove my rings. The gloves protect both my hands and my jewelry. ⤵

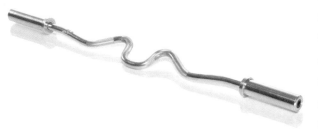

EZ-Curl Bars

When your arms are relaxed, your palms naturally face the body. EZ-curl (cambered) bars allow a more comfortable grip. They were created to make the curling exercise more natural, but now they are also widely used in close-grip bench pressing and flat overhead triceps extensions. EZ-curl bars are not superior to straight bars for curling, but they exercise different sets of muscle fibers. Periodically switching between cambered and straight bars will help stimulate your muscles.

Training Straps

Your grip frequently gives out before the larger muscles do in such exercises as dead lifts, chins, rows, pulldowns and shrugs. Training straps can actually enable you to perform several more reps. More reps means more progress. Training straps are usually made from strong cotton webbing or leather. ⤵

I usually use training straps when doing hanging leg raises — what a superb way to train abs!

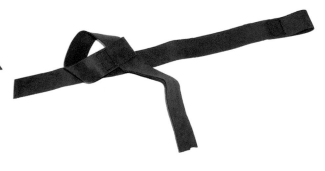

Heel Boards

Most people feel uncomfortable squatting with a weight if their feet are flat on the ground. A heel board (merely a piece of wood 2 ½ inches x 5 inches x15 inches) helps enable good squatting form. It also lessens the likelihood of strain to the Achilles' tendons, the soleus, and upper calf muscles. You have to get heel boards cut to size at a lumberyard.

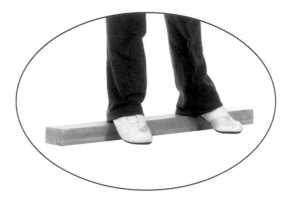

I never get over the thrill of walking into a well-equipped gym. The anticipation of the work that lies before me is just too exciting. I hope you feel this way too!

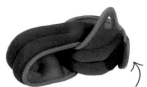

ankle & wrist weights

Ankle and Wrist Weights

Ankle and wrist weights make you work harder when doing cardio, thus benefiting the heart and lungs to a greater degree. Buy these items only if they are fully adjustable and can be fitted snugly to your limbs. Ankle and wrist weights can also be used for various abdominal leg lifts, but their use as progressive resistance is limited because the actual weight is limited. Be cautious, as some people have been known to injure their hip joints through improper use or overuse of ankle weights when running.

Dipping Belts

Once you reach the advanced level you may need more resistance on exercises such as parallel bar dips, chins and calf work. A dipping belt is then indispensable. Thread weight disks onto a chain attached to a dipping belt. Worn around the waist, this belt gives the body additional resistance. You can also get a weighted vest with pockets that serves the same purpose.

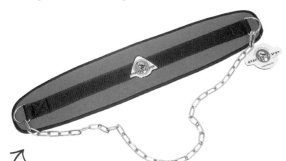

I have not progressed to this level myself but if you are a serious bodybuilder you may consider a dipping belt.

Lat Machines

This machine involves a pulley system of weight resistance. Lat machines are ideal for pulldowns (for the lats), and also pressdowns – an excellent movement for the triceps. Many lat machines are fitted with extra pulley wheels to redirect the basic resistance and allow for a greater variety of movements.

Olympic Barbell Springs

These unique items are used for quick changing of plates. They are squeezed into place, thus doing away with standard barbell collars, screws, and wrenches. They are not recommended for use with heavy dumbells.

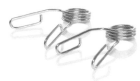

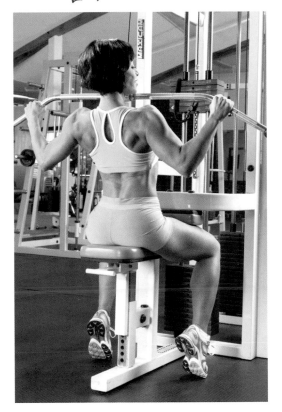

← Lat Machine

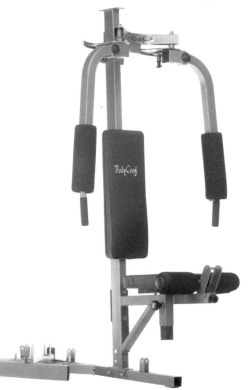

Pec-Decks

This apparatus was invented to improve the flye movement. The Pec-Deck is used in a seated upright position. Your arms begin straight out to the sides or bent upward. The movement involves the forward and inward motion of the arms, which places the stress exclusively on the pectoral muscles.

Multi-Purpose Benches

These benches are made in a variety of sizes and are available in all price ranges. The idea is to incorporate as many features as possible into one bench to accommodate the needs of trainers who do not have a great deal of room for equipment in their homes. Most multi-purpose benches include an adjustable incline bench, leg-curl and leg-extension attachments, weight stands, and flat-bench facilities. More expensive models include preacher benches, squat stands, dip bars, and even lat-machine attachments.

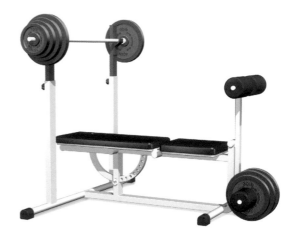

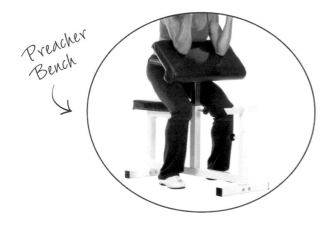

Preacher Bench

Preacher Benches

This is a special bench designed to keep the upper arms stationary and at an angle while the trainer curls any resistance. Preacher benches can be used in a standing or seated position. The angle of the padded bench surface is normally adjustable. Preacher benches are also known as Scott or Gironda benches.

Crossover Pulley Machines

This cumbersome machine is not considered a home unit because of its size. It enables the trainer to work the upper, middle, or lower pectoral muscles by simply raising or lowering the pulleys before performing the exercise. Crossover pulley machines also contribute to pectoral striations.

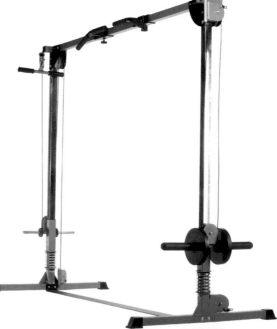

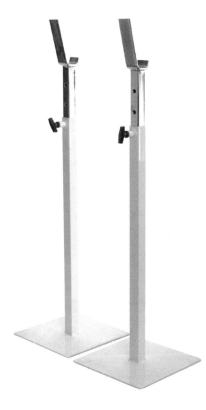

Squat Stands

Squat stands offer a way to train using heavy weights with utmost safety. The barbell is lifted from them prior to the squatting set and replaced after the set. They are not considered a home gym necessity, but if you are serious about training at home and want to make real progress in leg development, squat stands are important.

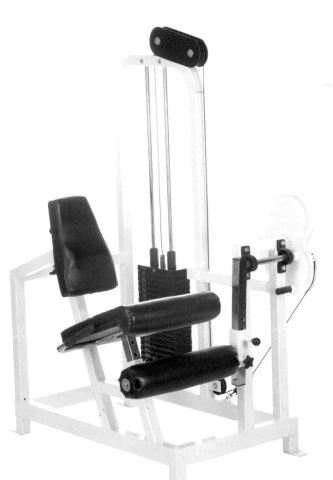

Leg-Extension Machines

A very popular apparatus because almost everyone is looking for a substitute for squats. The leg extension incorporates a padded seat with a roller bar attachment, enabling you to mobilize the leg muscles. Standing variations also exist.

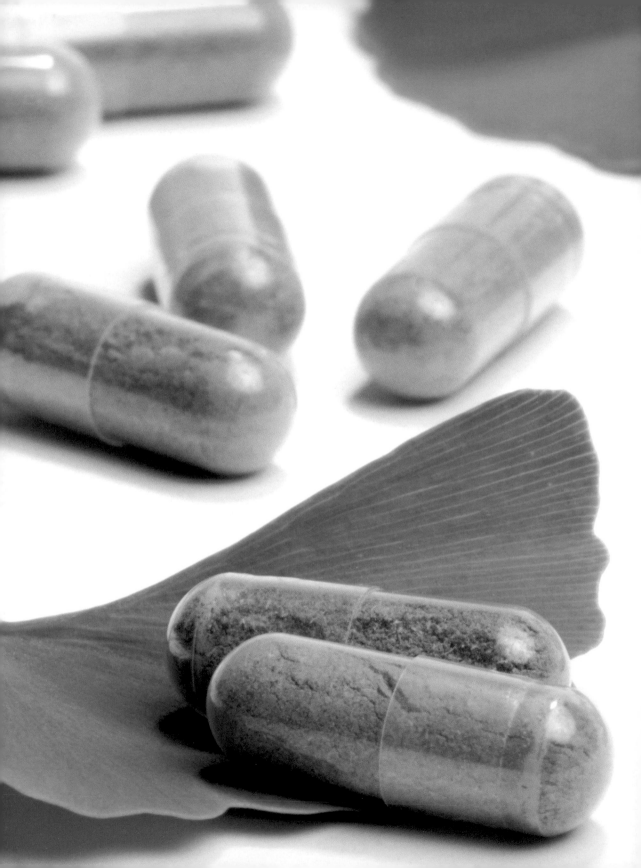

6

"Everything you put in your mouth takes its place inside your body. If your nutrition is of the highest, healthiest quality, so too will be your physique. Clean Eating takes the guesswork out of what to eat. Your body will glow with vitality once Clean-Eating magic takes place."

SUPPLEMENTATION
THE ADDED INGREDIENT

In today's stress-filled society, where our bodies have to cope with pollution, noise, and detrimental farming and food-transportation practices, supplementation is necessary for everyone. Even the addition of a multivitamin pill will make a positive difference.

Each vitamin has an RDA (Recommended Dietary Allowance), and those who eat a balanced diet filled with fresh, natural foods will reach these quotas. However, nutritional research has proven that the RDA allowances are far from adequate, and the optimal daily requirements are substantially higher, especially for those who exercise.

At times a woman may jeopardize the balance of her diet when bringing about physical changes. For example, a pre-contest diet may be low enough in calories to prevent adequate nutrition. She would be wise to offset any possible imbalance by taking a high-quality multivitamin/mineral pill daily.

Some is Better than Not Enough!

If a person is not getting the right amount of nutrition, she will not be able to function at her peak. No one knows this better than the Russians, whose athletes are regularly given hair or blood analysis tests to monitor their nutritional status. If the athlete is not getting enough iron, for example, this is quickly corrected with supplementation.

We should understand that supplements cannot work miracles. However, correct supplementation can put a woman at a tremendous physical advantage. More is not necessarily better when it comes to vitamins, but some is definitely better than not enough!

I am not suggesting that supplementation take the place of wholesome fresh food. Food always comes first. But you should consider supplementing your food intake with high-quality products to ensure that you are getting enough of what your body needs for top health, strength, condition and appearance. If you are getting inadequate nutrition, your results may be less than they could be.

Vitamins

Vitamins are not needed to produce energy – they are catalysts that "spark" the assimilation of other nutrients. They are essential in varying quantities as links in the metabolism of other nutrients to maintain efficient bodily function. No one food contains all the vitamins necessary for optimal growth and body maintenance.

Vitamins A, D, E and K (fat-soluble vitamins) can be stored in the body for short periods. Large dosages can be harmful, causing diarrhea and nausea. If you want to take high dosages of water-soluble vitamins such as the Bs and C, which *are* needed daily, take them separately to avoid excessive amounts of vitamins A and D.

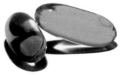

12 ESSENTIAL VITAMINS

VITAMIN A

For healthy bones, skin, teeth, resistance to infection, and good vision.

SOURCE: fish, eggs, dairy products, liver, tomatoes, quinoa, seaweed and sea vegetables, spinach, kale and carrots.

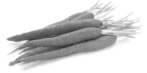

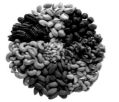

VITAMIN B1 (Thiamine)

For a healthy nervous system.

SOURCE: pork, organ meats (such as liver, kidney, and heart), whole-grain breads, cereals, peas, nuts, beans and eggs.

VITAMIN B2 (Riboflavin)

For the metabolism of proteins, fats and carbohydrates for energy and tissue building. It promotes healthy skin, particularly around the mouth, nose and eyes.

SOURCE: organ meats, liver, sausage, dairy, eggs, whole-grain breads, dried beans, and leafy green vegetables.

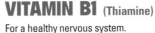

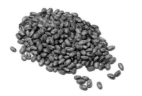

VITAMIN B4 (Niacin)

Promotes a healthy nervous system, healthy skin, aids digestion and helps cells use oxygen to release energy.

SOURCE: liver, meats, fish, whole-grain breads, dried peas and beans, nuts and nut butters.

VITAMIN B6 (Pyridoxine)

Aids in protein utilization and prevention of certain types of anemia. It is also helpful in maintaining normal growth.

SOURCE: liver, kidneys, butter, meats, fish, cereal, soybeans, tomatoes, peanuts, almonds and corn.

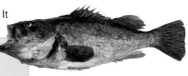

VITAMIN B5 (Pantothenic Acid)

Helps breakdown of fats, proteins and carbohydrates for energy.

SOURCE: organ meats, egg yolks, meats, fish, soybeans, peanuts, broccoli, cauliflower, potatoes, peas, cabbage and whole-grain products.

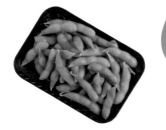

7 VITAMIN B9 (Folic Acid)

Promotes the development of red blood cells and the normal metabolism of carbohydrates, proteins and fats.

SOURCE: organ meats, asparagus, turnips, spinach, kale, broccoli, corn, cabbage, lettuce, potatoes and nuts.

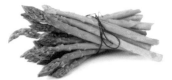

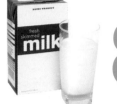

8 VITAMIN B12 (Cobalamin)

Produces red blood cells in bone marrow and builds new proteins. It also helps the normal functioning of nervous tissue.

SOURCE: liver, kidneys, lean meats, fish, hard cheese and milk.

9 VITAMIN C (Ascorbic Acid)

Helps bond cells together. It produces healthy teeth, gums and blood vessels, and improves iron absorption. It hastens the healing of wounds and improves resistance to infection. It also aids in the synthesis of hormones that regulate bodily functions.

SOURCE: citrus fruits (grapefruit, oranges, lemons), strawberries, cantaloupes, raw vegetables (especially green peppers), cauliflower, broccoli, kale, tomatoes, potatoes, cabbage, goji and acai berries, and brussels sprouts.

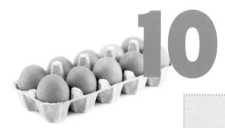

10 VITAMIN D

Promotes healthy bones and teeth and helps the body absorb calcium and phosphorus. There is a great deal of excitement around this vitamin lately, as researchers have found direct links to incidences of cancer and inadequate vitamin D.

SOURCE: liver, egg yolks, and foods fortified with vitamin D such as milk. It is also produced in the body by exposure to direct sunlight.

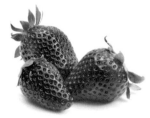

11 VITAMIN E

Protects red blood cells and slows destruction of vitamins A and C.

SOURCE: wheat-germ oil, rice, leafy green vegetables, nuts, margarine and legumes.

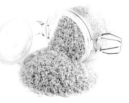

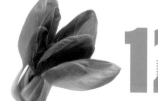

12 VITAMIN K

Permits blood clotting.

SOURCE: spinach, kale, cabbage, cauliflower and pork liver.

I strongly believe in consuming a variety of proteins, not just those from animal sources. Try vegetable protein from soy products and other plant-based proteins like quinoa and spirulina. For a great quinoa recipe check out Quinoa with Sundried Tomatoes in *The Eat-Clean Diet Cookbook.*

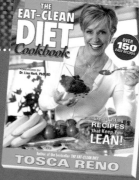

Minerals

Numerous minerals are required to maintain healthy bones and teeth, particularly calcium, while others aid in hormone production. Calcium is also utilized to maintain muscle tone and muscle recuperation after exercise, and it is partially responsible for heartbeat regulation. Other essential minerals include chromium, copper, fluorine, iodine, iron, magnesium, manganese, molybdenum, phosphorus, potassium, selenium, sodium and zinc.

Protein Supplements

Protein is needed to build muscle. In fact, a muscle is 10 percent protein – the rest is mostly water. However, the building blocks within the protein – amino acids – are of special concern.

The most recent findings show that most adults require no more than 0.37 grams of protein per pound of bodyweight per day. Children and teenagers, pregnant women, nursing mothers and athletes need more. Women trainers in need of added muscle size can certainly use extra protein, but massive amounts are unnecessary.

Hundreds of proteins exist. Each contains a different combination of amino acids. At least 20 amino acids have been identified so far, all but eight of which can be manufactured by the body. These eight are known as the essential amino acids, and they must come from food or supplementation.

Proteins can be used by the body to build muscle only if their proportions of amino acids are balanced

There is a multitude of protein supplements on the market. Check labels carefully for protein content and for sugar and added chemicals.

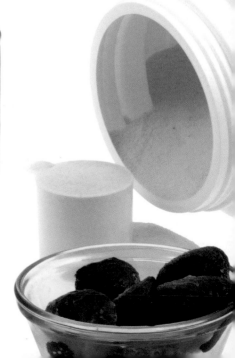

Eggs are a fantastic source of protein. They're one of the quickest ways to get your protein when you're in a rush.

correctly. This combination never seems to happen by itself in natural foods, which means no high-protein food can be fully utilized. The protein in eggs is closest to being complete — over 90 percent can be used. Dairy products, fish, meat, and poultry are also high on the list, with 60 to 80 percent of their protein usable. Grains, legumes, and vegetables are lower in usable protein, usually between 40 and 60 percent.

The fundamental function of protein is the maintenance and growth of tissue. If you are not getting enough, you will suffer loss of weight, have diminished resistance to disease, and you will get tired easily. On the other hand, continual large doses of protein over and above your requirements can actually be harmful to the body. It can cause calcium loss, weakening of the bones, and can even contribute to kidney problems and gout.

You'll find scores of bodybuilding and body-reducing supplements on the market. Look for quality. Are the protein-efficiency rations (PER) high? Do the products contain essential vitamins, minerals, amino acids and digestive enzymes? One advantage of supplementation is that you can feed your body added nutrients without necessarily increasing the energy content of your daily intake. This is particularly useful to a woman who is trying to peak for a specific event (wedding, school reunion, contest, etc.).

For those wanting to add muscle, weight-gain products can furnish high-quality nutrition and extra calories while lessening the burden of eating lots of food. These meals are also convenient. A nutrient-loaded shake is more fun to prepare than a formal meal. Read labels on all products. You don't want to be taking in more sugar or other no-no's such as trans fats. Beware especially of the sugar content in weight-gain products.

Keep this list handy!

GREAT SOURCES OF
PROTEIN

- Eggs and egg whites
- Lean meats, beef, pork
- Skinless chicken (white meat is leaner)
- Salmon, sole, halibut, cod, tilapia
- Soybeans, soy milk
- Low-fat dairy, skim milk, yogurt, cottage cheese
- Low-sugar protein powders
- Nuts, almonds, walnuts (watch your portions because nuts are high in good fats)

Steroids

Anabolic steroids are artificial derivatives of the male hormone testosterone. Men and women have hormones from both sexes in their bodies, but a man has considerably more testosterone than estrogen (the female hormone) and women have more estrogen than testosterone.

Unfortunately, some female athletes take anabolic steroids, which serve to make their bodies more masculine. They get stronger, more muscular and tend to shed fat more easily, especially in the hip and leg area, where many women have a tendency to store fat. Dangerous side effects can include increased hairiness, a deeper voice, aggressive behavior, diminishment of breasts, a premature aging of the muscle cells, and heart and organ problems, among others. Their impact on reproductive organs is unknown. I advise you not to take these for any purpose if you are healthy.

Innocent Beginnings

Steroids were developed in Germany to help people with muscle-wasting diseases. Today physicians routinely prescribe these potentially dangerous drugs … not to the sick, but to the healthy. They are dished out to runners, cyclists, field athletes, tennis pros, football players, weightlifters,

"I don't know about you, but I much prefer the look of a toned female physique with some muscle to the look of a muscle-bound man-woman!"

The sooner we close the chapter on steroid abuse, the better off all sports will be.

golfers, bodybuilders and basketball and baseball players in staggering quantities.

Women were first accused of using steroids almost a half-century ago. Suspicion was initially prompted by the masculine appearance of some of the Russian Olympic athletes in track and field. By the mid '70s women were definitely linked with taking steroids – first track and field athletes, then powerlifters, and now, in ever-increasing numbers, women in almost every sport. Very few will admit it. Although I am vehemently against the use of steroids by both sexes, a woman taking artificial male hormones is particularly unwise. Steroids are illegal drugs. There is definitely an aspect of ignorance associated with women who take steroids – if they knew the potential dangers surely they would not take them.

Steroids and Fitness

Fitness women who have been in the sport a number of years tend not to resort to drug use. However, those new to fitness competition often can't wait for natural results. Many try steroids almost from the beginning because they want their bodies developed overnight. Almost 30 percent of women competing are estimated to be using anabolic steroids.

In women's fitness contests, points are awarded for the degree of proportionate muscle size, and for low body-fat levels and well-defined ("ripped") muscles. These results can be obtained the healthy way – from steady, progressive training and Clean Eating. Do not play Russian roulette with anabolic steroids.

All sports suffer from the steroid connection. Even though the majority of competitors, and almost all non-competitors, do not take drugs, the word is out that the more muscular women do take them. Athletic organizations are taking strong stands against them. The sooner we close the chapter on steroid abuse, the better off all sports will be. In case I haven't made myself clear: Steroids kill!

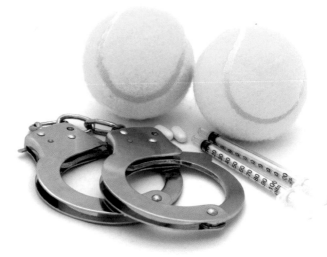

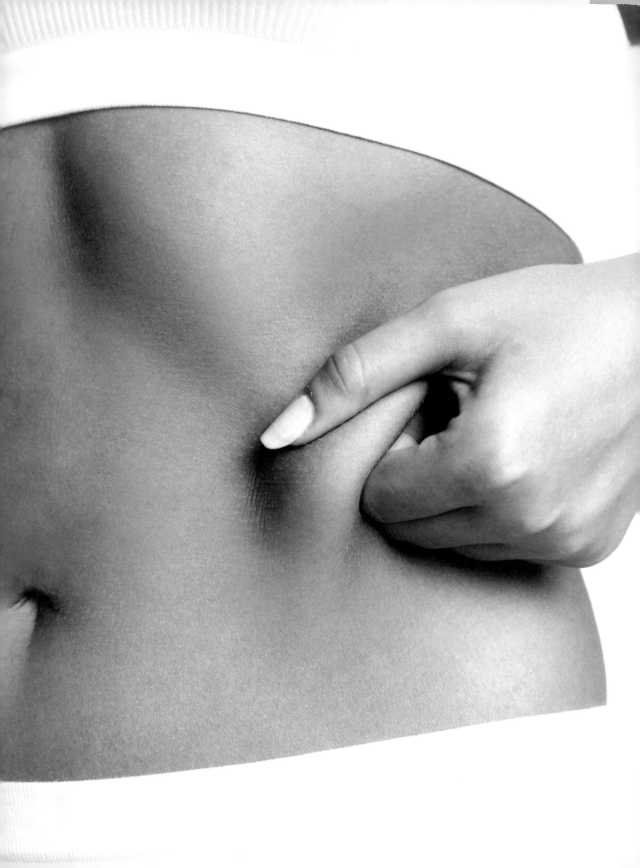

7

"Clean Eating and weight training changed my life in such a stunning way. I am certain this is the way life is supposed to be lived. Don't let one more day go by burdened by excess weight or poor health. Make this your first day of being the best you ever."

THE LEAN ADVANTAGE
LOSING EXCESS FAT

You may be 30, 40 or even 150 pounds overweight. Or perhaps you just want to shed 5 to 10 pounds. Whatever the case, the strategy is the same.

Many diet books, pills and programs state that you do not need to have willpower or that there is no need to control portions. This is all baloney. Losing weight takes conscious effort.

Why are you overweight right now? According to Dr. Stuart Berger, "The basic causes of being overweight, whether 2 or 200 pounds, are almost always psychological." Perhaps your mother fed you every time you cried as a baby. As a child you might have been rewarded with a chocolate bar or a box of cookies if you were upset. There is no doubt

that oral stimulation (eating) provides quick relief for emotional distress.

We may use food as an oral "pacifier." It comforts us even as it makes us fat. Being fat often builds its own emotional upset. If we see ourselves as unattractive we may withdraw from social relationships. This gives us a sense of emptiness and depression, which we fight by overeating. We are trapped in a vicious circle.

The key to weight reduction is diet and Clean Eating is the way to go. Never make the mistake of cutting your calorie intake in half. Drastic cuts are just not workable. Neither is fasting. Both practices put your body in shock. Besides, cutting off your food supply in a drastic manner simply doesn't work as well

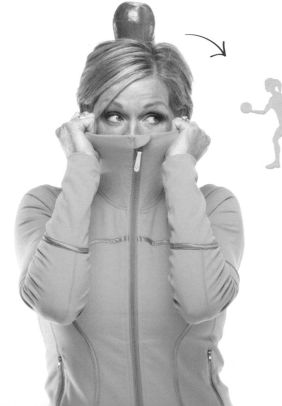

TIP

Don't hang all your hopes for weight loss on a pill. Doing so will only leave you frustrated once again and in danger of gaining more weight. Rely only on your own inherent power and on this book for guaranteed results.

as you may imagine. Invariably the body reacts by bracing itself for the famine, storing extra fat on which to live. Many scientific studies have shown

> **Once you have a balanced diet of fruits, vegetables, whole grains, poultry, lean-meat, fish, and skim-milk products, you can carry on the gradual reduction of overall junk calories consumed while still keeping a balanced food intake.**

that harsh, unbalanced diets or fasts actually cause the body to become fatter. More fat-depositing enzymes are produced and create what Covert Baily, the author of *Fit or Fat*, describes as "the fat person's chemistry, " a *tendency to get fat.*

Your diet can be cleaned up in stages. You don't need to be drastic. Start by dropping added sugar and candy from the diet, then reduce all calorie-dense snacks, such as chocolate. Next remove potato and corn chips, cakes, cookies, and butter. Get all the junk foods out. Once you have a balanced diet of fruits, vegetables, whole grains, poultry, lean-meat, fish, and skim-milk products, you can carry on the gradual reduction of overall junk calories consumed while still keeping a balanced food intake.

Aerobic Exercise – Fat as Fuel

Food intake is key, but aerobic exercise also helps with weight reduction. Weight training is considered an anaerobic activity (without oxygen), although a

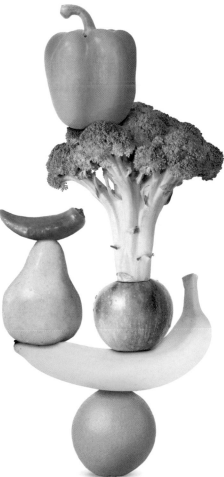

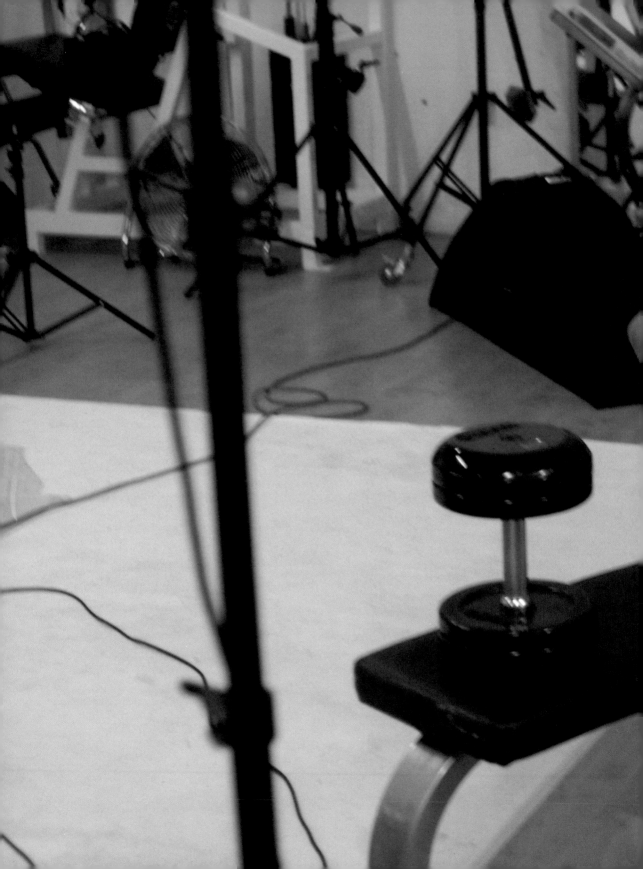

My little secret is: I don't spend hours in the gym. I incorporate physical activity into my day in any way I can . . . even at a photo shoot!

person could get an aerobic effect by increasing the pace in her weight workouts. Aerobic activities are of low to moderate intensity and should be continued for a minimum of 20 minutes. The beauty of aerobic exercise is that energy comes from the body's store of fat.

Aerobics, or cardio, should be practiced three or four times each week. Exercise that requires 80 percent or less of your maximum heart rate is considered aerobic. If you push your heart to higher than 80 percent of its maximum (as is often the case with vigorous weight training), then the exercise is anaerobic. To find out an estimate of your maximum heart rate, subtract your age from 220. Then multiply by .80 to learn the heart-rate threshold between aerobic and anaerobic activity. Moderately paced swimming or brisk walking are aerobic activities because they keep your heart well below 80 percent of maximum rate (Refer to page 30 for a complete target heart-rate zone chart).

A Lifestyle Change

Once you have normalized your bodyweight with aerobic exercise and Eating Clean, do not allow yourself to develop bad habits again. Your aim should be to maintain low body fat for the rest of your life! In the early stages, this may prove to be difficult, because you will have to eliminate all of those bad eating habits that created the excess fat to begin with.

I think of this as a revised attitude towards food, a lifestyle change. I want you to understand fully that your eating habits in the past were unacceptable. They must be revised. Understand your true need for wholesome, unadulterated foods, and eat small portions five or six times each day. This may sound like a tall order. All I can say is: Master it and you will be putting yourself in line for a longer, healthier, fitter, pain-free existence of self-contentment and joy.

Muscles on Women?

The world's greatest artists throughout history have paid homage to the beauty of the female body. From the ancient Venus de Milo, now in the Louvre Museum in Paris, to the work of modern artists today, the form of the feminine physique has been represented by those with the ability to transcribe shape to canvas or marble. And then came women's fitness.

TIP
"I rarely view exercise as something I have to do. Rather, I think of it as something I have the privilege to do"

Not long ago the question was asked in the UK: "How would you like your ideal man to look? Would you like him ripped to shreds with an amazing six-pack? Should he be moderately built with a small paunch? Or should he be 60 pounds overweight and built like a truck driver?" The answer came back three to one. Women (of the UK at least) wanted to be comfortable with their man who possessed a reasonably small paunch (a potbelly no less) over the male six-pack image!

Ten years ago North American women were asked in an *Oxygen* magazine survey what they thought about women with abdominal muscles that clearly showed as defined ridges in their midsection. The answer came back loud and clear. The vast majority of women hated the thought of having defined abs. And remember, these were subscribers to *Oxygen*, a women's fitness magazine!

How things have changed! Today, women admire the abs of fitness stars Monica Brant, Maggie Diubaldo and Alicia Marie, while show biz stars like Janet Jackson, Pink and Madonna are worshipped for their abs as much as their voice.

Proportionate and Toned

Whether at this stage you want visible abs or not is immaterial. I'm sure you want a proportionate, toned and balanced physique, and that is what I plan to give you. I tell you with every honest fiber of my being: You can do it! Fat or thin, tall or short, young or not so young, you can change your physique and enjoy a brand new healthy lifestyle just as I have done.

How? Follow a two-edged program of Eating Clean (to reduce the fat) and weight training (to tone and shape the muscles). Throw in a little cardio, and you're good to go. Yes, it takes courage to start. It takes dedication and perseverance. But hey, you can start today! And as sure as eggs are eggs, if you keep at it your body will change. Fat will disappear, tone will arrive and your shape will show your beauty off to the world. Remember when you were young and didn't realize how gorgeous you were? Well, you're going to get that back. I came back from being a 40-year-old housewife, locked into an unhappy relationship, to being in the best shape of my life. I got myself a new attitude, a new body, new energy, new health and a lifestyle of daily joy.

We have to keep in mind that weights and diet are tools that can work magic, but you must use these tools sensibly. Don't make the common mistake of thinking that because your upper arms are flabby and your waist is thicker than it should be, that you only need a few triceps exercises and some crunches. In every case, you need to work the entire body. None of us reach absolute perfection, but my training plan coupled with Clean Eating will make you the healthiest, fittest and most beautifully put together woman you can be!

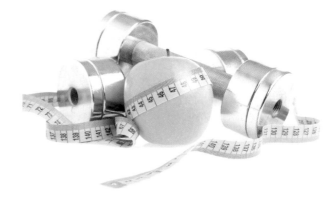

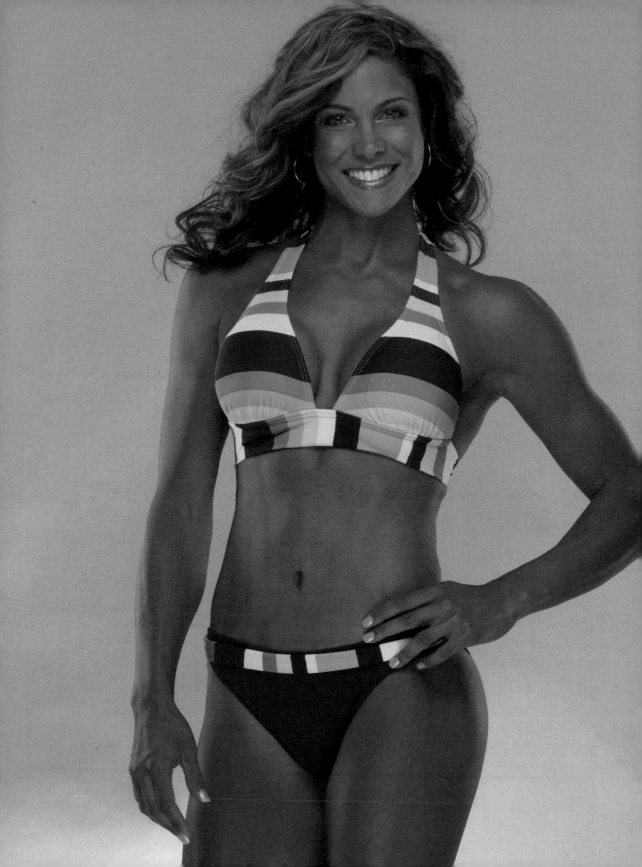

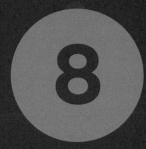

8

"Owning a layer of taut muscle tissue is a surefire way of increasing your metabolic rate and banishing fat tissue from your body."

IDEAL PROPORTION
MUSCLE WHERE IT COUNTS

The essence of fitness training is to develop balanced proportion. This applies to men as well as women. But somehow the women seem to better understand this idea than men. Men will spend hour upon hour, day upon day, working their biceps and chest, yet neglect all their other muscles. I have yet to meet a female gym member who isn't aware of her proportion, or lack thereof. When her body is not in perfect harmony she is worried, and certainly women spend a great deal of time trying to attain balance.

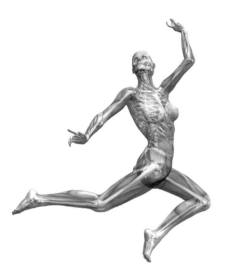

Balanced proportion does not just occur by itself. You have to first think about it, then plan for it and subsequently train for it. Like a sculptor or architect, you must always be aware of what you're doing. You must work for physical balance.

The late Vince Gironda, who not only trained himself to prize-winning shape but was also a trainer to the stars

of stage and screen (including Marilyn Monroe), said: "Although a muscle has four sides, and each aspect has to be trained, that does not mean that you should train each part of a muscle equally hard." In other words, in the name of visual perfection we should train our weak points hard and put less effort into areas that are already toned and developed.

Let's talk briefly about each body part, detailing how you can utilize the correct training approach to create the best results. Most women are aware of the effect that clothes have on their appearance. Puffy sleeves will do wonders for rounded, small shoulders. Well-cut pants make hips look slender. High-heeled shoes create an illusion of longer legs.

Just as you can use clothes to hide or accentuate certain body parts, you can tailor your muscles to highlight your overall physique. Add a bit here; take away a bit there, and presto! Before you know it, your complete dynamic physique is emerging.

HERE ARE SOME TIPS:

Shoulders

Build the side (lateral head) if you are too narrow in this region. Dumbell lateral raises will do the job. If your shoulders are rounded or drooping forward, then incorporate plenty of dumbell bent-over raises and bent-over rows in your workout to work the rear head (posterior deltoid).

I was able to create mobility in my scapulae and widen the flair of my back even at the age of 40 by working hard at "pulling out" my lats.

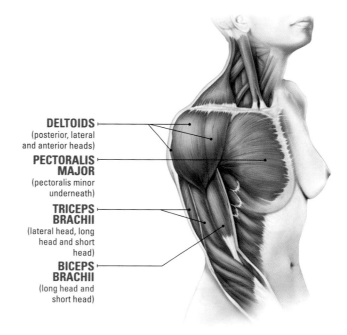

DELTOIDS
(posterior, lateral and anterior heads)

PECTORALIS MAJOR
(pectoralis minor underneath)

TRICEPS BRACHII
(lateral head, long head and short head)

BICEPS BRACHII
(long head and short head)

Chest

It is important to fully develop the outer areas of the pectoral muscles to accentuate the V-shape flair of the torso. This is done with wide-grip parallel bar dips (if you can do them), and incline and flat-bench flye exercises with dumbells. Wide-grip bench presses also develop this area.

Biceps

The best exercises for developing the peak of the biceps are the 45-degree incline dumbell curl and the preacher-bench curl with the pad set at 90 degrees (vertical). Working the lower biceps is accomplished by setting the preacher bench at a shallow angle of about 25 degrees (almost horizontal).

Triceps

If you build up your triceps high near the deltoid (shoulder), your arm will appear to taper from the shoulder to a diminishing elbow region. It is more aesthetically pleasing to have the upper-arm muscles gradually tucking neatly into the elbow region.

A good exercise for the lower triceps region is the single-arm triceps extension in the seated or standing position. Another good one is the standing close-grip barbell (or EZ-curl bar) extension behind the head, holding the elbows as close to the ears as possible. The best lower triceps movement is the dumbell kickback (with your torso and upper arm parallel to the floor).

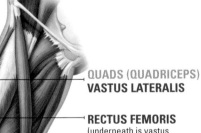

GLUTES
GLUTEUS MEDIUS
GLUTEUS MAXIMUS
(gluteus minimus underneath)

HAMSTRINGS
SEMITENDINOSUS
BICEPS FEMORIS
SEMIMEMBRANOSUS

GASTROCINEMIUS
(calves – inner & outer)

SOLEUS

QUADS (QUADRICEPS)
VASTUS LATERALIS

RECTUS FEMORIS
(underneath is vastus intermedius)

VASTUS MEDIALIS

Calves

Need more development of the outside of the calves? Then do your heel-raise exercises with the toes pointing inward. Development on the inside of the calf is achieved by performing your calf raises with your toes pointed outward. For best overall shape of the lower leg, exercise with your bodyweight mainly on the big toe.

Unfortunately, many women are limited by lack of mobility in the ankle joint. For best results, you must use as full a range of motion as possible, which means going upwards and downwards all the way. I have had to work diligently on this limitation of mine as I have naturally small calves. Sigghhhh!!

The bottom part of the lower leg (the soleus) is exercised by utilizing the seated calf-raise machine.

Thighs

The upper quads (rectus femoris and vastus lateralis) and glutes are worked with squats and lunges. Lower quads (vastus medialis) are brought into play when the body leans rearwards during squatting movements, as with hack squats and sissy squats. Leg extensions build cuts into the thighs, while leg curls build the hamstrings.

TIP

Abs can take a lot of punishment — training them three or four times per week to exhaustion is not too much.

Lats

The lats (short for latissimus dorsi), being the largest back muscles and those most responsible for that dramatic V-taper, should be worked hard to improve their flair. This taper is arrived at not just by building the lats, but also by stretching out the scapula (the shoulder blades). Wide-grip chins and pulldowns contribute to this desired result.

If you want to develop more of the lower lat area (careful now – too much lower lat can ruin your V-taper), then do plenty of bent-over rows and seated cable pulls, always pulling the handles toward the waist area.

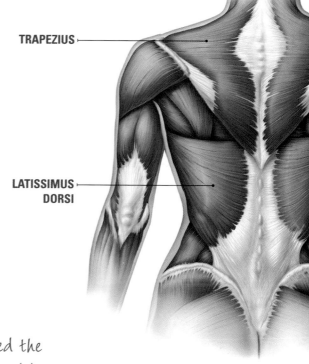

TRAPEZIUS

LATISSIMUS DORSI

TIP

The ideal shape to strive for is called the "wild physique," a shape characterized by broad shoulders, narrow hips and waist, sweeping quads and small knees.

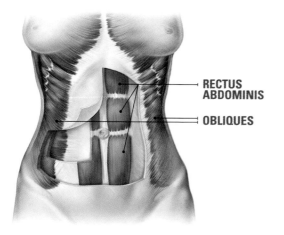

RECTUS ABDOMINIS

OBLIQUES

Abdominals

In the old days it was quite acceptable if a fitness contestant showed only a couple of rows of abdominal muscles to the judges. Today she needs abs above and below the navel.

The hanging leg raise is the best exercise for the lower abs. Another good exercise is the reverse crunch, whereby the legs are lowered below the hips in each repetition and the butt is lifted off the bench at the top of the movement. This is one of my favorites for targeting those hard-to-isolate lower abs.

Posture

Good posture is important for everyone. It is achieved when all the elements of the body are balanced vertically on each other. The word "posture" indicates the manner in which we carry the body when standing, sitting or walking. You change posture every time you change your activity. That posture change can be either correct or lazy. It's easy to develop poor posture, especially if your job is sedentary, and if you practice bad posture long enough it becomes habitual. The same is true of good posture. Practice it and it can become an integral and graceful part of you.

Although an upright stance is a natural position, most people droop and become round shouldered, especially older people. To avoid this "stoop," make a constant effort to correct your posture throughout the day. Once you get the hang of it, proper posture will become second nature. Curiously enough, those who think they are relaxing by slouching are actually causing added fatigue to set in.

A woman who stands well – upright and proud – holds within her a beauty asset. In his book *Exercise*, Dr. Herbert M. Shelton states: "Erect carriage is exceedingly important to the health and vigor, as well as the best appearance, of man and woman." Poor posture can result in stress and strain, causing discomfort and pain.

THESE ARE COMMON POSTURAL MALADIES:

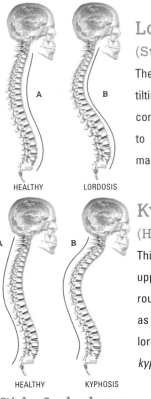

HEALTHY   LORDOSIS

HEALTHY   KYPHOSIS

Lordosis
(Swayback)

The abnormal forward tilting of the pelvis. This condition contributes to general abdominal malfunctions.

Kyphosis
(Humpback)

This results when the upper back is overly rounded. Combined, as it often is, with lordosis, it is called *kyphlordosis.*

Side Imbalance

Disturbed lateral balance of the spinal column gives unequal shoulder height (one is lower than the other). This can result from one leg being shorter than the other or from a tilted pelvis, but more often than not it results from poor habits, such as sitting with one leg under the other (which causes abdominal weakness and curved upper back).

Certain postural malfunctions are beyond immediate control, but most are preventable and remediable. Most can be corrected by postural awareness and by regular practice of corrective exercises.

HERE ARE A FEW CORRECTIVE EXERCISES FOR SPECIFIC PROBLEMS.

DROOPING HEAD

Sit upright in a chair, with your chin touching your upper chest. Clasp your hands behind your head and push your head back while resisting strongly with your hands. Do 1 set of 15 repetitions.

ROUND SHOULDERS

Sit with hands clasped behind your head, keeping your back and head in a straight line. With hands behind your head, spread your elbows as far back as possible, tightening the upper-back muscles to their limit. Do this exercise every day for 1 set of 10 repetitions.

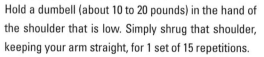

UNEVEN SHOULDERS

Hold a dumbell (about 10 to 20 pounds) in the hand of the shoulder that is low. Simply shrug that shoulder, keeping your arm straight, for 1 set of 15 repetitions.

Few exercises in themselves will correct poor posture. Sports or athletic pursuits can help slightly, but some sports even contribute to severe postural defects. Judo and figure skating cause lower-back hollowness. Cycling can round upper backs. Weight training helps because all muscles are involved, helping you build healthy core strength.

Remember, postural improvement will result from overall strengthening exercises plus constant attention to correcting your stance whenever you catch yourself slouching or drooping. Severe postural problems should, of course, be addressed with your doctor.

Scuptural Balance

Weight training is not a haphazard pastime. When a woman sets out to build and shape her body, it makes sense for her to build muscle only in the areas where it will look attractive and add to her overall balance. You are restyling your entire physique – sculpting it, if you will. Do it right from the start and you won't have to undo any of your hard work later.

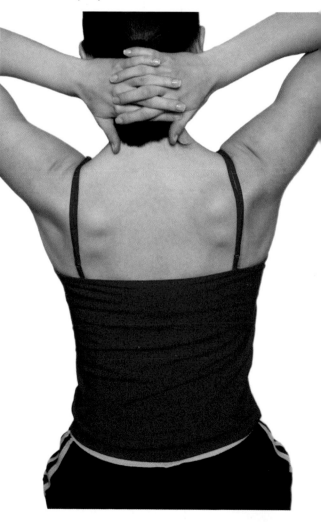

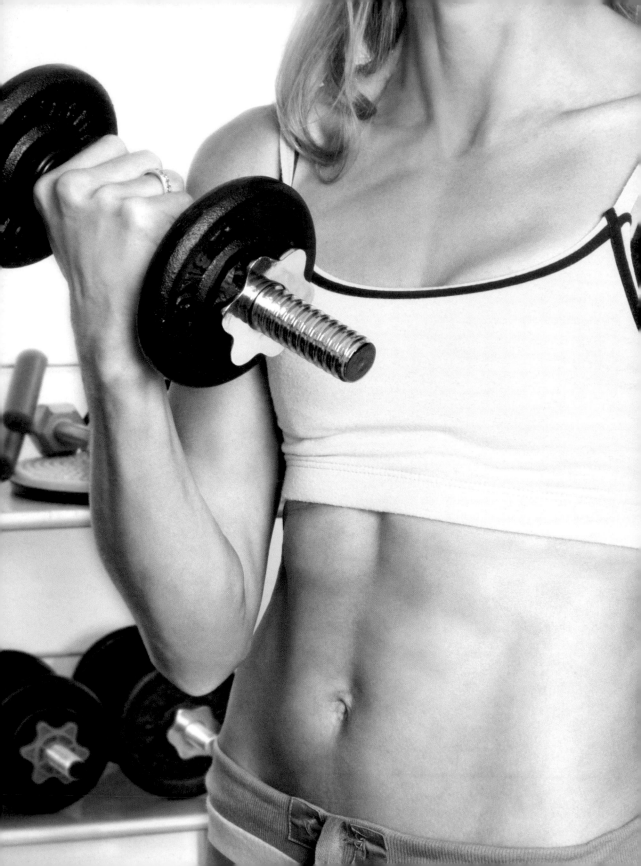

9

"The new language of barbells, dumbells, weight stacks, squats, presses and lunges helped me gain a profound awareness of the 600 or more muscles in my body that sorely needed work. When I started lifting, Muscle Magic happened in short order. I want you to experience it, too."

YOUR WORKOUT ROUTINE
PUTTING IT TOGETHER

You have many important points to consider when creating your routine. Before you put pen to paper and write out your own physique renovation routine, consider the following recommendations.

EXERCISE ALL BODY PARTS.

Even if you feel that your upper body and arms are pretty good and that you need to work only your legs and waistline, work your whole body. It is a big mistake to think that you need to exercise only certain body parts and not all. That does not mean you have to work every body part every workout (though you could), but just as part of your weekly schedule.

DO NOT MAKE YOUR ROUTINE TOO LONG.

You have to work within your ability to recuperate and within the capacity of your energy level. If your routine is too short, you may not be exercising all major body parts. A too-long routine causes overtraining, which is worse. Overtraining has a negative effect on the body and will ultimately lock you into a plateau, or sticking point. In extreme cases it weakens the body's immune system, making you more susceptible to viruses and other sickness.

PERFORM EXERCISES WITH A SPECIFIC GOAL.

Don't waste your time squatting if your upper thighs are already too big and muscular. Forget heavy lateral raises if your shoulders are already wide enough.

Do specific peak exercises if you have no biceps height. Do more lower abdominal work if you have little muscularity in that area. You must tailor your exercises to your specific aims. In my case I had to spend a lot of time developing my V-taper. That translated into loads of back work, improving the mobility of my scapula, and trimming my waist.

DO A WORKABLE WORKOUT FREQUENCY.

The well-tested guideline is to work each muscle two or three times a week. If you train any particular muscle once a week or less, then beyond a certain point you will likely not continue to make progress. On the other hand, if you train a body part too often it cannot recuperate properly.

You will recall that you can train your whole body three times a week, or you can do various "splits," depending on your ability and schedule.

Training frequency can get a little complicated. Not everyone can train when he or she wants. Some gyms are not open on Sundays and some of us have shift work, overtime, school hours or family obligations that do not always fit in easily with training requirements. You just have to do the best you can in difficult circumstances. Where there's a will there's a way. Can you make progress by training each body part just once a week? In a word: yes. Though this is not optimal, it's better than not training at all.

Included in the next few pages are a selection of weight routines for you to try. The multitude of weight-training information can be overwhelming so I have broken it down for you into beginner, intermediate and advanced options. I myself have used these tried-and-true routines and have included my journal excerpts for you to see. You can follow the exact programs as listed in my journal or modify them to fit your lifestyle and training needs. Remember, these routines are guidelines only! These are the weights I used, but they may not be ideal for you, so adjust them according to your strength. To create your own workout journal please use the tear-outs found at the back of the book.

Let's get started!

THE BEGINNER'S ROUTINE

It is probably best for the beginner to train three times a week with one rest day between each workout. Do not try to use heavy weights at first. Perform your exercises in good (strict) style. Complete beginners should perform only one set of each exercise, but after a few weeks you should be able to do two or three sets.

BEGINNER:
TOSCA'S BEGINNER ROUTINE

DATE *Feb 12, 1999*

BODY PART	EXERCISE		SET 1	SET 2	SET 3	SET 4	SET 5
Thighs	Squats	WEIGHT	30lbs				
		REPS	10				
Chest	Bench Presses	WEIGHT	10lbs				
		REPS	8				
Upper Back	Wide-Grip Lat Pulldowns	WEIGHT	30lbs				
		REPS	10				
Triceps	Lying Triceps Extensions	WEIGHT	30lbs				
		REPS	10				
Biceps	Barbell Curls	WEIGHT	10lbs				
		REPS	8				
Abs	Crunches	WEIGHT	∅				
		REPS	15				

CARDIO ACTIVITY:

Warm Up — 10 minutes of walking outside. I did my 1st step class yesterday. It was awesome! I felt really energized afterwards.

NOTES:

Today was my first day of weight training. I got oriented with the equipment and ready to go. It was great! I feel powerful and strong. I can't wait for the next session.

THE STRENGTH-BUILDING ROUTINE

Strength-training routines are traditionally short because the number of available exercises is limited. You work the large muscles when training for overall power. Strength training means more sets, fewer reps, and more rest time between heavy sets (up to two minutes).

INTERMEDIATE:
TOSCA'S STRENGTH-BUILDING ROUTINE

DATE *May 9, 2003*

BODY PART	EXERCISE		SET 1	SET 2	SET 3	SET 4	SET 5
Chest	Bench Presses	WEIGHT	45lbs	55lbs	70lbs	85lbs	55lbs
		REPS	10	10	10	10	25
Thighs	Squats	WEIGHT	Ø	60lbs	115lbs	165lbs	115lbs
		REPS	15	12	8	6	10
Shoulders	Presses Behind the Neck	WEIGHT	35lbs	55lbs	45lbs	45lbs	45lbs
		REPS	8	8	8	10	12
Lower Back	Dead Lifts	WEIGHT	45lbs	45lbs	45lbs		
		REPS	11	11	11		
Upper Back	Bent-Over Rows	WEIGHT	45lbs	75lbs	85lbs	85lbs	75lbs
		REPS	8	9	10	8	10

CARDIO ACTIVITY:

Warm Up — 5 minutes of jump rope. I did a yoga class last night with my daughter. It was very relaxing and much needed.

NOTES:

This routine is a long one and pretty tiring so I made sure I had a great breakfast this morning, complete with my favorite oatmeal pancakes and a delicious egg-white omelet. It was the perfect start to my day and I had a ton of energy to get through my workout.

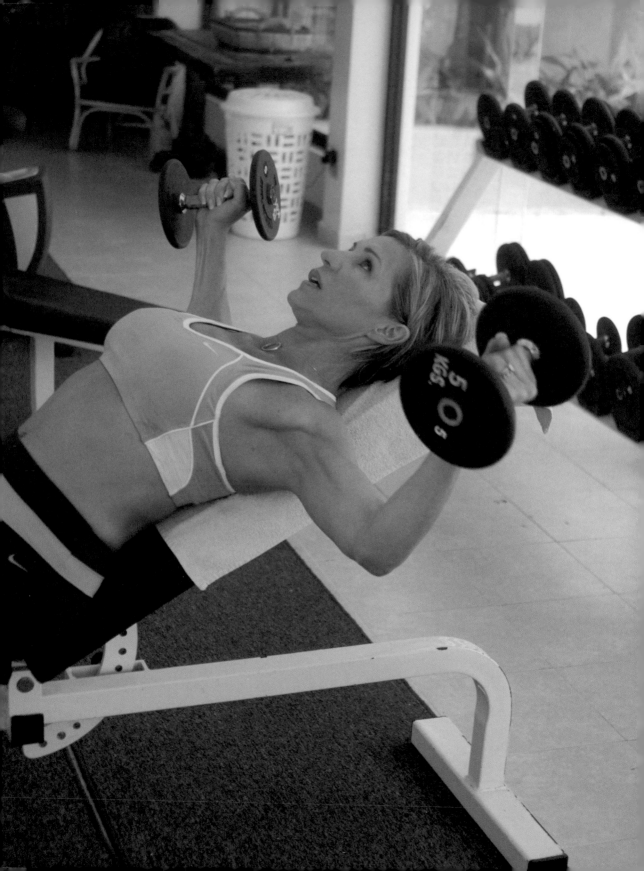

THE SHORT ROUTINE

Obviously, you must make every effort to get a quality workout in a short period of time, but use caution so as not to get injured! Each exercise here has two sets. Your first one must still act as a warm-up set. For the second set you must put forth a maximum effort.

INTERMEDIATE:
TOSCA'S SHORT ROUTINE

DATE Jan 21, 2003

BODY PART	EXERCISE		SET 1	SET 2	SET 3	SET 4	SET 5
Chest	Bench Presses	WEIGHT	55lbs	80lbs			
		REPS	15	15			
Upper Back	Lat Pulldowns	WEIGHT	70lbs	120lbs			
		REPS	12	12			
Shoulders	Upright Rows	WEIGHT	45lbs	55lbs			
		REPS	15	15			
Thighs	Leg Presses	WEIGHT	200lbs	300lbs			
		REPS	12	12			
Triceps	Close-Grip Bench Presses	WEIGHT	35lbs	45lbs			
		REPS	12	15			
Biceps	Incline Dumbell Curls	WEIGHT	10lbs	15lbs			
		REPS	12	15			
Forearms	Wrist Curls	WEIGHT	10lbs	10lbs			
		REPS	15	15			
Calves	Standing Calf Raises	WEIGHT	90lbs	165lbs			
		REPS	25	25			
Abs	Bench Crunches	WEIGHT	Ø	Ø			
		REPS	45	55			

CARDIO ACTIVITY:

Circuit Training (done twice) — 1) running stairs for 5 minutes 2) jump rope for 5 minutes 3) jog for 5 minutes – this circuit kept my energy high and my interest piqued — I'll definitely do it again!

NOTES:

I was really busy today and for half a minute considered not working out at all. But a short workout is infinitely better than none! I'm glad I did it.

THE BASIC ROUTINE

As the name implies, this routine works the basic muscle groups. It is abbreviated, yet adequate as a maintenance routine. Because the sets are limited, I advise you to do a high-intensity workout. Push hard at the end of the set, especially the last set of each exercise. Be sure, however, to maintain good exercise form.

INTERMEDIATE:
TOSCA'S BASIC ROUTINE

DATE Oct 10, 2002

BODY PART	EXERCISE		SET 1	SET 2	SET 3	SET 4	SET 5
Chest	Bench Presses	WEIGHT	60lbs	85lbs	85lbs		
		REPS	8	8	8		
Upper Back	Bent-Over Rows	WEIGHT	50lbs	70lbs	70lbs		
		REPS	10	10	10		
Thighs	Squats	WEIGHT	60lbs	110lbs	120lbs		
		REPS	10	10	10		
Shoulders	Seated Dumbell Presses	WEIGHT	15lbs	20lbs	25lbs		
		REPS	8	8	8		
Calves	Standing Calf Raises	WEIGHT	100lbs	120lbs	120lbs		
		REPS	25	25	25		
Biceps	Barbell Curls	WEIGHT	30lbs	40lbs	40lbs		
		REPS	10	10	10		
Triceps	Lying Triceps Extensions	WEIGHT	30lbs	40lbs	45lbs		
		REPS	12	12	12		
Abs	Reverse Crunches	WEIGHT	Ø	Ø	Ø		
		REPS	20	20	20		

CARDIO ACTIVITY:

Warm Up — 10 minutes of stair climbing.
I really needed a good warm up today. Fall has finally hit and it's one of those days that chills you right to the bone.

NOTES:

I'm back to the gym after a weekend of visiting my family. I stuck to my Clean Eating and took lots of walks while I was away, but I missed the weights. My training session was welcome today!

TIP

TIP

This is the time to train smarter, not longer. I love that about weight training. Specific trouble spots get more attention.

THE MUSCLE-ISOLATION ROUTINE
(UPPER/LOWER SPLIT)

This type of workout results in increased separation between individual muscles. They show up more as individual units. Use lighter weights and provide direct stress to a single muscle or muscle group.

ADVANCED

DATE Feb 4, 2004

TOSCA'S MUSCLE-ISOLATION ROUTINE
DAY 1 (UPPER BODY)

BODY PART	EXERCISE		SET 1	SET 2	SET 3	SET 4	SET 5
Chest	Dumbell Flyes	WEIGHT	15lbs	20lbs	25lbs	25lbs	
		REPS	12	12	12	12	
	Pec-Deck Flyes	WEIGHT	60lbs	60lbs	70lbs	70lbs	
		REPS	12	12	12	12	
Upper Back	Single-Arm Rows	WEIGHT	40lbs	50lbs	60lbs	60lbs	
		REPS	10	10	10	10	
Shoulders	Lateral Raises	WEIGHT	15lbs	15lbs	20lbs	20lbs	
		REPS	10	10	10	10	
	Incline Rear Laterals	WEIGHT	10lbs	10lbs	15lbs	15lbs	
		REPS	12	12	12	12	
Triceps	Single-Arm Lying Triceps Extensions	WEIGHT	10lbs	10lbs	12lbs		
		REPS	12	12	12		
	Standing Triceps Extensions	WEIGHT	20lbs	30lbs	30lbs		
		REPS	12	12	12		
	Lying Triceps Extensions	WEIGHT	20lbs	30lbs	30lbs		
		REPS	10	10	10		
Biceps	Preacher-Bench Curls	WEIGHT	20lbs	30lbs	40lbs		
		REPS	10	10	10		
	Single-Arm Pulley Curls	WEIGHT	20lbs	30lbs	30lbs	30lbs	
		REPS	12	12	12	12	
Forearms	Wrist Curls	WEIGHT	20lbs	20lbs	20lbs		
		REPS	15	15	15		
	Reverse Wrist Curls	WEIGHT	15lbs	20lbs	20lbs		
		REPS	15	15	15		

CARDIO ACTIVITY: Warm Up — jump rope for 5 minutes

NOTES: Today was my 1st day of the muscle-isolation program. I'm getting started on show preparation and will be tightening up my diet soon.

TIP

If it's safe to do so, I will sometimes touch the muscle I am working with my free hand while performing the exercise. This helps me put my mind into the muscle – give it a try!

ADVANCED

DATE Feb 5, 2004

TOSCA'S MUSCLE-ISOLATION ROUTINE
DAY 2 (LOWER BODY)

BODY PART	EXERCISE		SET 1	SET 2	SET 3	SET 4	SET 5
Thighs	Leg Extensions	WEIGHT	60lbs	80lbs	100lbs	120lbs	100lbs
		REPS	10	10	10	8	10
	Leg Curls	WEIGHT	60lbs	60lbs	80lbs	80lbs	
		REPS	12	12	12	12	
Calves	Standing Calf Raises	WEIGHT	100lbs	120lbs	140lbs	200lbs	200lbs
		REPS	20	20	20	20	20
	Seated Calf Raises	WEIGHT	50lbs	60lbs	90lbs	90lbs	
		REPS	20	20	20	20	
Abs	Crunches	WEIGHT	Ø	Ø	Ø	Ø	
		REPS	25	25	25	25	
	Hanging Leg Raises	WEIGHT	Ø	Ø	Ø	Ø	Ø
		REPS	20	20	20	20	20

CARDIO ACTIVITY: Running on treadmill for 35 minutes
— 5.5 mph, 2.5 incline

NOTES: I'm really feeling Day 1 in my muscles, but I'm still energized. Today's workout was a hard one, too. I love that sweet pain in my muscles, but I'm looking forward to a rest day tomorrow!

THE HEAVY AND LIGHT ROUTINE
(PUSH/PULL SPLIT)

There are benefits from training both heavy and light. You maximize muscle tone, separation, and build both muscle fiber and capillary size. Additional fiber size and strength result from using the heavier weight; tone, endurance, and pump comes from the lighter work.

ADVANCED
DATE April 4, 2005

TOSCA'S HEAVY AND LIGHT ROUTINE
DAY 1 (PUSH)

BODY PART	EXERCISE		SET 1	SET 2	SET 3	SET 4	SET 5
Chest	Bench Presses	WEIGHT	80lbs	80lbs	90lbs	100lbs	100lbs
		REPS	5	5	5	5	5
	Incline Dumbell Flyes	WEIGHT	20lbs	20lbs	20lbs	20lbs	
		REPS	15	15	15	15	
Thighs	Squats	WEIGHT	100lbs	120lbs	140lbs	160lbs	160lbs
		REPS	5	5	5	5	5
	Leg Extensions	WEIGHT	40lbs	60lbs	80lbs	80lbs	
		REPS	15	15	15	15	
Shoulders	Dumbell Presses	WEIGHT	20lbs	25lbs	30lbs	30lbs	30lbs
		REPS	6	6	6	6	6
	Lateral Raises	WEIGHT	15lbs	15lbs	15lbs	20lbs	
		REPS	15	15	15	15	
Calves	Standing Calf Raises	WEIGHT	140lbs	140lbs	150lbs	180lbs	200lbs
		REPS	10	10	10	10	10
	Donkey Calf Raises	WEIGHT	∅	∅	∅	∅	
		REPS	20	20	20	20	
Triceps	Parallel Bar Dips	WEIGHT	∅	∅	∅	∅	∅
		REPS	5	5	5	5	5
	Triceps Pressdowns w/rope	WEIGHT	30lbs	45lbs	45lbs	50lbs	
		REPS	15	15	15	15	

CARDIO ACTIVITY: Warm Up — stair climbing for 5 minutes

NOTES: I'm a few weeks into this heavy and light program and it was time to increase my weight for each exercise. I'm going to have a good protein smoothie now to help my muscles recover.

TIP
The heavy and light routine targets fast-twitch muscle fibers that predominate in quick, powerful movements, and slow-twitch muscle fibers that are important for slow, maintained movements.

ADVANCED
DATE April 5, 2005

TOSCA'S HEAVY AND LIGHT ROUTINE
DAY 2 (PULL)

BODY PART	EXERCISE		SET 1	SET 2	SET 3	SET 4	SET 5
Upper Back	Barbell Rows	WEIGHT	60lbs	70lbs	80lbs	80lbs	80lbs
		REPS	5	5	5	5	5
	Lat Pulldowns	WEIGHT	50lbs	60lbs	60lbs	60lbs	
		REPS	20	20	20	20	
Biceps	Barbell Curls	WEIGHT	50lbs	60lbs	60lbs	60lbs	
		REPS	6	6	6	6	
	Pulley Curls	WEIGHT	30lbs	30lbs	30lbs	30lbs	
		REPS	15	15	15	15	
Abs	Weighted Roman Chair	WEIGHT	10lbs	20lbs	20lbs		
		REPS	10	10	10		
	Seated Bent-Knee Tucks	WEIGHT	Ø	Ø	Ø		
		REPS	30	30	30		

CARDIO ACTIVITY: I love cardio day! I took the dogs for a run today for 30 minutes up and down a hill. It was tough, but I feel great now!

NOTES: I had a delicious omelet this morning at breakfast. I added some fresh rosemary from the garden. I have to make it again soon. My family loved it!

THE BACK-SPECIALIZATION ROUTINE
(TWO-DAY SPLIT)

The back needs to be exercised from various angles because of the many different muscles involved – the rhomboids, teres, latissimus dorsi, trapezius, and erector spinae. As with all specialization programs, begin your routine with the area you want to develop.

ADVANCED
TOSCA'S BACK SPECIALIZATION
DAY 1

DATE Sept 29, 2006

BODY PART	EXERCISE		SET 1	SET 2	SET 3	SET 4	SET 5
Back	Wide-Grip Chins	WEIGHT	Ø	Ø	Ø	Ø	
		REPS	10	10	10	10	
	Bent-over Rows	WEIGHT	60lbs	70lbs	70lbs	80lbs	80lbs
		REPS	8	8	8	8	8
	Wide-Grip Pulldowns	WEIGHT	80lbs	100lbs	120lbs		
		REPS	12	12	12		
	Narrow-Grip Pulldowns	WEIGHT	100lbs	120lbs	140lbs		
		REPS	12	12	12		
	Incline Dumbell Rows	WEIGHT	30lbs	30lbs			
		REPS	10	10			
	Prone Hyperextensions	WEIGHT	Ø	Ø			
		REPS	15	15			
Calves	Standing Calf Raises	WEIGHT	120	160	180		
		REPS	20	20	20		
Abs	Reverse Crunches	WEIGHT	Ø	Ø	Ø		
		REPS	35	35	35		

CARDIO ACTIVITY: Warm Up – 5 minute jog outside

NOTES: Today's not cardio day, but I did a great HIITs routine yesterday. I've been noticing some weakness in my back so I tried out this back-specialization routine. I've split it between 2 days.

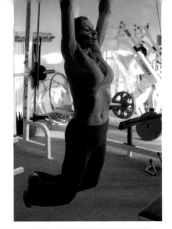

ADVANCED
TOSCA'S BACK SPECIALIZATION
DAY 2

DATE Sept 30, 2006

BODY PART	EXERCISE		SET 1	SET 2	SET 3	SET 4	SET 5
Chest	Incline Bench Presses	WEIGHT	40lbs	40lbs	50lbs		
		REPS	10	10	10		
Shoulders	Seated Dumbell Presses	WEIGHT	20lbs	25lbs	25lbs		
		REPS	8	8	8		
Thighs	Squats	WEIGHT	100lbs	130lbs	160lbs		
		REPS	8	8	8		
	Leg Curls	WEIGHT	60lbs	80lbs	80lbs		
		REPS	12	12	12		
Triceps	Standing Triceps Extensions	WEIGHT	25lbs	30lbs	30lbs		
		REPS	12	12	12		
Biceps	Alternate Dumbell Curls	WEIGHT	15lbs	20lbs	20lbs		
		REPS	8	8	8		

CARDIO ACTIVITY: *Warm Up — 10 minute jog outside — I have to take advantage while the weather is still warm!*

NOTES: *I am really feeling yesterday's back workout. Glad to know it's working! I really have to work on my weak areas.*

THE CHEST-SPECIALIZATION ROUTINE
(TWO-DAY SPLIT)

Because this routine focuses on the chest, the pectoral exercises are grouped at the beginning of the workout.

Notice that we start with the heavier chest exercises and finish with the pec-isolation movements.

ADVANCED
TOSCA'S CHEST SPECIALIZATION
DAY 1

DATE Mar 15, 2007

BODY PART	EXERCISE		SET 1	SET 2	SET 3	SET 4	SET 5
Chest	Bench Presses	WEIGHT	60lbs	80lbs	100lbs	120lbs	80lbs
		REPS	8	8	8	8	8
	Incline Dumbell Presses	WEIGHT	25lbs	25lbs	30lbs	30lbs	30lbs
		REPS	8	8	8	8	8
	Parallel–Bar Dips	WEIGHT	Ø	Ø	Ø		
		REPS	8	8	8		
	Cross–Bench Dumbell Pullovers	WEIGHT	25lbs	30lbs	30lbs		
		REPS	12	12	12		
	Dumbell Flyes	WEIGHT	20lbs	25lbs	25lbs		
		REPS	12	12	12		
	Pec–Deck Flyes	WEIGHT	30lbs	40lbs	50lbs		
		REPS	12	12	12		
Erectors	Good Mornings	WEIGHT	20lbs	30lbs	30lbs		
		REPS	15	15	15		
Abs	Bench Crunches	WEIGHT	Ø	Ø	Ø		
		REPS	40	40	40		

CARDIO ACTIVITY: Warm Up — 5 minutes jump rope

NOTES: My daughter joined me for my workout today. We had a jump rope competition for 5 minutes. She blew me out of the water! But I showed her on this chest routine!

TIP

Keep your workouts the correct length for you. Too short and you won't get the job done; too long and you'll still feel tired when you rise in the morning.

ADVANCED
TOSCA'S CHEST SPECIALIZATION
DAY 2

DATE Mar 16, 2007

BODY PART	EXERCISE		SET 1	SET 2	SET 3	SET 4	SET 5
Thighs	Leg Presses	WEIGHT	200lbs	250lbs	300lbs		
		REPS	10	10	10		
	Leg Curls	WEIGHT	60lbs	80lbs	80lbs		
		REPS	12	12	12		
Shoulders	Upright Rows	WEIGHT	30lbs	50lbs	50lbs		
		REPS	10	10	10		
Upper Back	Close-Grip Lat Pulldowns	WEIGHT	80lbs	120lbs	120lbs		
		REPS	12	12	12		
Triceps	Triceps Pressdowns	WEIGHT	40lbs	60lbs	60lbs		
		REPS	12	12	12		
Biceps	Preacher-Bench Barbell Curls	WEIGHT	30lbs	50lbs	50lbs		
		REPS	10	10	10		
Forearms	Behind-Back Wrist Curls	WEIGHT	20lbs	30lbs	30lbs		
		REPS	15	15	15		
Calves	Seated Calf Raises	WEIGHT	50lbs	90lbs	90lbs		
		REPS	20	20	20		

CARDIO ACTIVITY: I ran on the treadmill for 35 minutes at 6 mph and 2.5 incline. I just put a bunch of new songs on my iPod so I was really energized.

NOTES: I think it's time to switch up my program. I'm getting a little bored after a few weeks of this routine even with new music! I'll sub in some new exercises next time.

THE LEG-SPECIALIZATION ROUTINE
(UPPER/LOWER SPLIT)

"Specialization" means that you put more effort into additional exercises for a specific body area. It does not mean that you stop working the other body parts. You still exercise them with a moderate amount of work. Because you are trying to improve one section of your body (an underdeveloped section) more than the others, you should perform these exercises first in your routine, since you have a high energy level and can give your best to the exercises.

ADVANCED
TOSCA'S LEG SPECIALIZATION
DAY 1 (LOWER)

DATE Dec 5, 2006

BODY PART	EXERCISE		SET 1	SET 2	SET 3	SET 4	SET 5
Thighs	Squats	WEIGHT	120lbs	160lbs	180lbs	200lbs	
		REPS	8	8	8	8	
	Leg Presses	WEIGHT	200lbs	250lbs	300lbs		
		REPS	10	10	10		
	Leg Extensions	WEIGHT	90lbs	100lbs	120lbs	120lbs	
		REPS	12	12	12	12	
	Leg Curls	WEIGHT	80lbs	90lbs	100lbs	100lbs	
		REPS	12	12	12	12	
	Lunges	WEIGHT	30lbs	40lbs	50lbs		
		REPS	12	12	12		
	Sissy Squats	WEIGHT	Ø	Ø			
		REPS	20	20			
Calves	Standing Calf Raises	WEIGHT	140lbs	160lbs	200lbs	200lbs	
		REPS	20	20	20	20	
	Seated Calf Raises	WEIGHT	60lbs	80lbs	90lbs		
		REPS	20	20	20		
	Donkey Calf Raises	WEIGHT	Ø	Ø	Ø	Ø	
		REPS	20	20	20	20	

CARDIO ACTIVITY: Warm Up — 5 minutes of jump rope

NOTES: I'll be starting my competition prep in a few weeks and I really need to work on my "skinny" chicken legs...haha... I tried this routine to get the ball rolling.

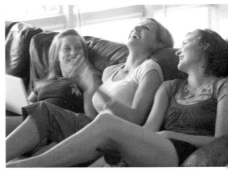

TIP

In the beginning I fought the idea of resting during the day. Now I see it as a moment to recuperate and get caught up on some reading or chatting with my family. You need to take a rest!

ADVANCED
TOSCA'S LEG SPECIALIZATION
DAY 2 (UPPER)

DATE Dec 6, 2006

BODY PART	EXERCISE		SET 1	SET 2	SET 3	SET 4	SET 5
Chest	Bench Presses	WEIGHT	60lbs	60lbs	60lbs		
		REPS	10	10	10		
Shoulders	Upright Rows	WEIGHT	40lbs	50lbs	50lbs		
		REPS	10	10	10		
Upper Back	Single-Arm Dumbell Rows	WEIGHT	40lbs	50lbs	50lbs		
		REPS	8	8	8		
Biceps	Barbell Curls	WEIGHT	40lbs	50lbs	60lbs		
		REPS	8	8	8		
Triceps	Triceps Pressdowns	WEIGHT	60lbs	60lbs	60lbs (v-bar)		
		REPS	12	12	12		
Forearms	Wrist Curls	WEIGHT	20lbs	30lbs	30lbs		
		REPS	15	15	15		
Abs	Hanging Leg Raises	WEIGHT	Ø	Ø	Ø		
		REPS	20	20	20		

CARDIO ACTIVITY: 10-minute jog. Wow! I overdid my leg workout yesterday and had to take a day off of cardio to give them some more recovery time.

NOTES: Next day I'll add another ab exercise. I don't think one is enough for this split routine. I'll add crunches next time.

The Recovery Factor

After vigorous weight training, the muscle cells must have rest time and nourishment to achieve recuperation. If you continually rework your muscles before they have properly recovered from the previous workout you will never make noticeable gains.

For the best results, train your body hard and then rest long enough that you will recover completely by your next workout. How do you feel the morning after a workout? Alive and ready to rise to any demanding challenge, or tired and physically drained?

A slight degree of soreness in the muscles means they are in the process of recuperating. I like this feeling because it is a reminder of the work I did the previous day. I embrace that Sweet Pain. If the soreness is extreme, however, then you have overdone it and recuperation will take longer.

There is a fine line between stimulating your muscles and overtraining. You may stimulate your muscles into growth or added tone with more sets, more intensity, or by switching to new exercises or combinations of exercises. If you push too hard, however, your muscles won't have time to recuperate. Overtrained muscles often appear flat and stringy, and body fat becomes difficult to shed.

How can we speed up recuperation? Read the following advice.

Spend a few minutes, two or three times a day, breathing deeply in the great outdoors.

Relaxation

When you rest, the body is in an ideal state to mend itself quickly. Try to put your legs up at least once a day and read a book or watch television. Hobbies can help you to relax. Do whatever appeals to you most. Of course, you don't actually have to do anything. Why not take a nap? I like that idea!

Stress is not beneficial to the body's recuperation system. If you've ever experienced severe stress or strain, you know how debilitating it can be. Our digestive system shuts down, our heart and breathing rhythms falter, and adrenaline and other hormones surge throughout the body. Momentarily we are at a peak for some type of physical action (fight or flight), but ultimately we become deflated and exhausted. If this happens regularly then our training progress will not amount to much and our overall health will decline.

Fresh air and sunshine are helpful. We hear so much about the sun causing skin cancer, but there would not be one speck of life on earth if it weren't for the sun. A prolonged lack of sunlight can cause rickets and contribute to other physical disorders. Spend a few minutes, two or three times a day, breathing deeply in the great outdoors. You will energize your entire physique. However, avoid sunburn. Exposure to the sun is good, but burning the skin is damaging to your health and excessive sun can be deadly.

Clean Eating

If you push your muscles to the limit, you can't expect them to recuperate unless they are fed correctly. You need at least the RDA of protein, vitamins, and minerals. I suggest you take multivitamins, and you might also benefit from taking an additional vitamin B complex, vitamins C and E, and some type of chelated mineral supplement.

You may discover that your recuperation is poor while you are trying to slim down or prepare for a special event. You have probably reduced your complex carbohydrates to a level too low for muscle recuperation. Take in more vegetables, brown rice and whole grains to beat the problem before it beats you. Eat to reach physique perfection, not near starvation.

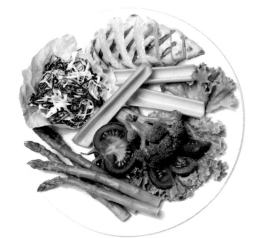

TIP

Clean Eating is the only healthy way to maintain your ideal body weight.

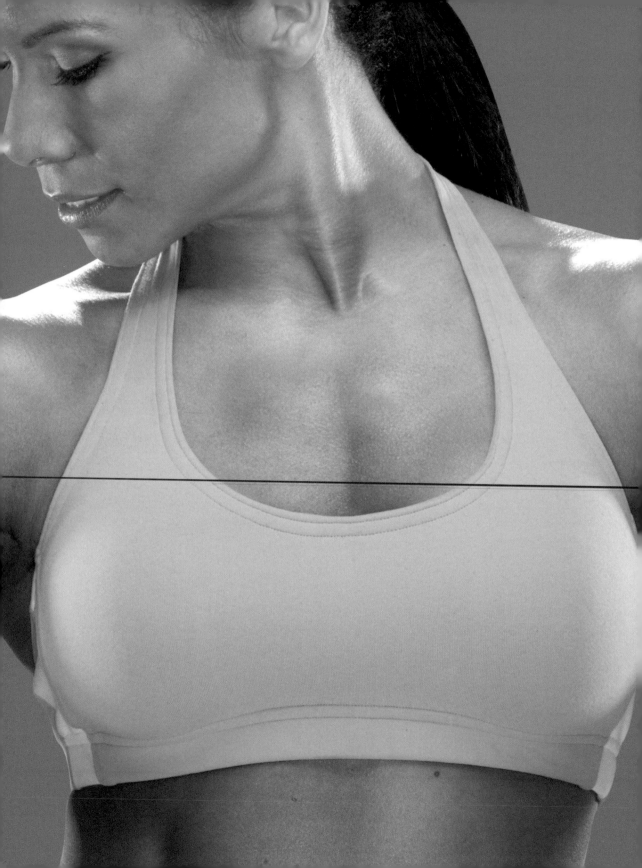

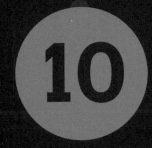

Delete all images of muscle-bound he-men from your mind! A strong chest is nothing but sexy. Working your pecs will even give you an instant bust lift — nice!

CHEST
BUILDING THE PECTORALS

Women are sometimes a little over-enthusiastic about developing the muscles in their chest. Some advanced trainers even go so far as to perform 20 to 30 sets of exercises for this body part. This is far too heavy a workload and would lead to a severe case of overtraining in all but the most seasoned trainers. It's better to train smarter, not harder.

The granddaddy of all exercises for the chest area is the most favored and famous movement of them all – the bench press! I love the feeling of powering up the weight as I lie beneath it. The way you perform this exercise will alter the results:

You can use different hand spacing. A shoulder-width grip works the inner pecs, while a wide grip works the outer pecs.

You can vary the spot on the chest to which you lower the bar. (Lower it to the sternum or breast bone to develop the lower chest. Lower it to the neck or collarbone area for the upper chest.) If you choose to lower the weight to an area of the chest between the two extreme points, then the area at which the bar touches the chest is the part that is exercised most.

The bench press is a beautiful exercise. You lie on your back, face up. Nothing moves but your arms. You feel very stable and relaxed. At first you may find some difficulty in balancing the bar, but after a while you find your groove and no longer have to consciously think about the mechanics of the movement.

I should mention that breasts cannot be enlarged by exercise. Weight training builds the underlying muscles of the chest and it can help lift the breasts but not increase their size. If you want larger breasts, this will come about from overall weight (fat) increase, taking birth control pills, or from implants. A word of warning – women with breast implants cannot perform heavy chest exercises. Heavy chest

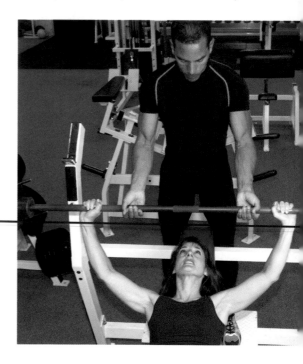

training can cause the implants to travel outwards to the side of the rib cage. Not a pretty sight at all and much more common than you think.

Although the bench press should form the basis of your chest workout, you should probably include at least one other exercise for the chest area. Dumbell flyes and presses give a good stretch. Pullovers work the middle and upper chest and expand the rib cage. Incidentally, you cannot *significantly* enlarge the rib cage with any exercise. If you are born with a shallow rib cage, then no amount of stretching, deep breathing, squats, or pullovers will change it significantly.

By the same token, a deep barrel chest cannot be made smaller. Ribs and other bones do grow to accommodate additional weight and decrease when the bodyweight is lost, but these changes are minimal. The human skeleton, after normal growth has ended, does not have a huge capacity for change.

If you admire the well-defined look that top fitness women get in their upper chests, do plenty of isolation moves in your chest routine. Exercises such as strict incline flyes and pec-deck flyes (push the forearms together at the end of each rep!) will do the trick. "Remember, though," says fitness expert Dr. Lynne Pirie. "Maximum striations only come when you have really peaked your body by restricting your food intake."

When sculpting your chest, bear in mind that all incline exercises work the upper chest; while decline (head lower than body) exercises train the lower pectorals. Parallel bar dips also work the lower chest muscles, but if the dip bars are set farther apart, say 22 to 30 inches (55 to 75 cm), depending on your height (the taller you are the wider apart the bars should be), then you will strongly activate the important outer pectorals.

As with other exercises, use the weight correctly as a tool to achieve your goal. Here is fitness star Monica Brant's opinion on this subject: *"You are not in a bench-press contest. The goal is not so much to get the weight up as it is to push with the isolated strength of the muscles you are training."*

Always remember to stretch the pectorals fully. After your first warm-up sets you can fully extend the motion. Dumbells generally permit more of a stretch than the barbell.

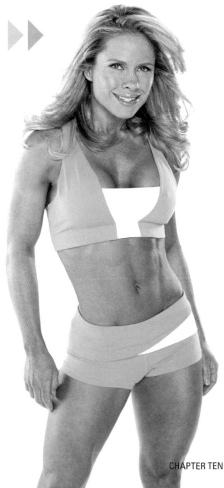

BENCH PRESSES

Overall Pectoral Area ▷ ▷ ▷ ▷
(6-12 REPS EACH SET)

Lie face up on a bench. Take a grip, thumbs under and around the bar and hands about two feet (60 cm) apart. Your forearms will be vertical when your upper arms are parallel to the floor. (This is the perfect hand distance).

Lower the weight from the straight-arm position to the pectorals. Touch the bar lightly on the chest (no bouncing) and press upward. Keep your elbows under the bar, and don't allow them to come close to the body.

Beginners may find that the bar starts to fall either forward or backward, or that the weight rises unevenly because one arm is stronger than the other. Time and practice will cure these minor faults.

Don't allow the bar to drop to your chest! Always control its descent deliberately. You could crack your sternum if the weight drops too rapidly.

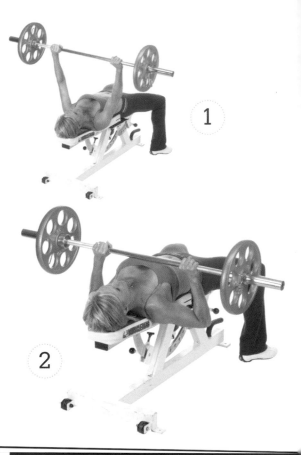

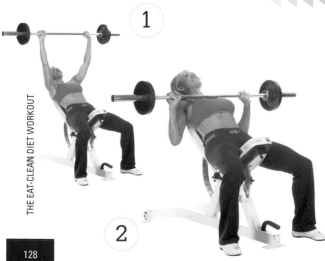

INCLINE BENCH PRESSES

Upper Chest
(8-12 REPS EACH SET)

◁ ◁ ◁ ◁

Start by lying on an incline bench set at a 35- to 40-degree angle. (More than 40 degrees will put too much emphasis on the front deltoids.) Press the barbell straight up, lock the elbows, and immediately lower the weight to the starting position. Keep the up-down movement going without pause. Your head should face up throughout the exercise. Keep your feet flat on the ground and do not arch your body as you press the weight up.

THE EAT-CLEAN DIET WORKOUT

SUPINE FLYES

Outer Pectorals ▷▷▷▷
(10-12 REPS EACH SET)

Years ago this exercise was done very rigidly with light weights, since the experts of the day insisted that the arms be fixed in a straight position. Today we still insist on a fixed position, but one in which the arms are bent as though they were in a plaster cast. This takes the strain off the elbow joint, allows more weight to be used, and gives you greater control and even better-toned chest muscles!

While lying face up on a bench with your feet planted firmly on the ground, lift the dumbells and then lower them to the side. Really go for the stretch once your muscles are warm.

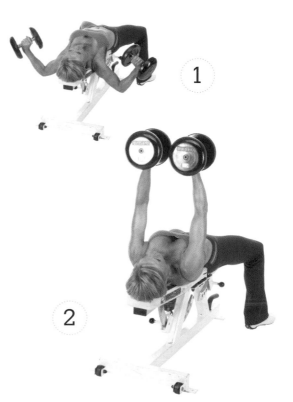

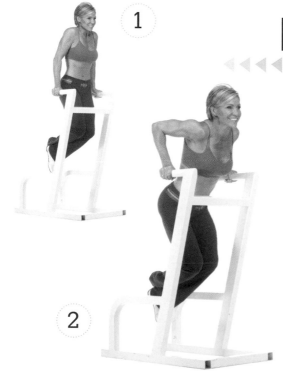

PARALLEL BAR DIPS

◁◁◁◁ Lower and Outer Pectorals
(8-20 REPS EACH SET)

This is a wonderful chest movement, especially if the bars are set fairly wide apart – 22 to 30 inches (55-75 cm). Narrow-set parallel bars will promote more triceps (upper arm) activity, but will still work the lower and outer pectorals. Wide-set parallel bars will benefit the upper-outer part of the chest. This development will make you look wide in the upper torso and shoulders. In other words, your V-taper will improve. Lower yourself as far as possible and lock your elbows as you straighten up.

INCLINE FLYES
Upper and Outer Chest ▶ ▶ ▶ ▶
(8-12 REPS EACH SET)

Adopt a secure position on an incline bench (a 30- to 40-degree angle is best). Hold up a pair of light dumbells, and then allow your arms to lower slowly out to the sides. Keep your elbows locked in a slightly bent position throughout the exercise. Lift and lower slowly, keeping the weights under control as each repetition stretches the chest. Keep your feet firmly planted on the ground. Resist the temptation to arch your back.

1

2

1

2

FLAT DUMBELL BENCH PRESSES
◀ ◀ ◀ ◀ Overall Chest
(8-10 REPS EACH SET)

Lie on your back on a flat bench; face up, feet firmly on the floor. Take one dumbell in each hand and, starting at the chest level with palms facing forward, press the dumbells simultaneously to the straight-arm position above the chest.

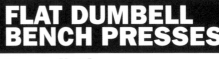

CROSS-BENCH DUMBELL PULLOVERS

Upper and Middle Pectorals ▶ ▶ ▶ ▶
(10-15 REPS EACH SET)

Lie across a flat exercise bench, holding a single dumbell with both hands (thumbs around the bar, fingers touching the inside plate).

Keeping your arms slightly bent, lift the weight from behind your head to above your chest and back down again. This exercise helps to mobilize the rib cage. Use a light weight when beginning this exercise.

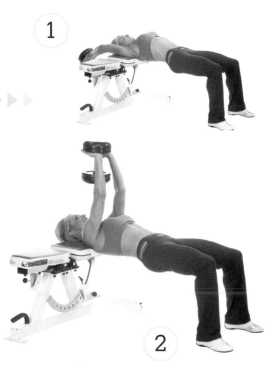

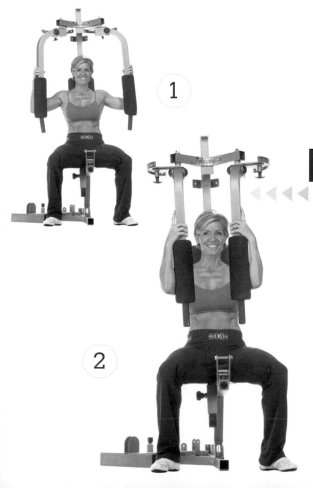

PEC-DECK FLYES

◀ ◀ ◀ ◀ Overall Chest
(10-15 REPS EACH SET)

A pec-deck is a large apparatus found in most gyms, the function of which is to almost exclusively work the pectoral muscles (although some people adapt the apparatus to work the rear deltoids by sitting in the opposite position).

Hold the "grippers" as indicated and bring your arms together in front of your chest by contracting the pectorals. Return to the starting position.

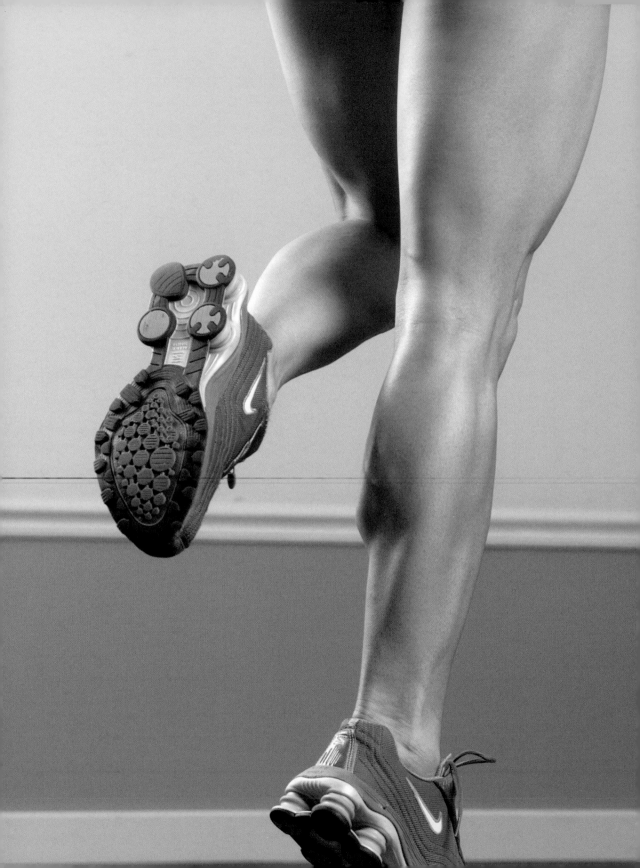

11

Chicken legs and cankles are no contest when faced with a no-fail weight-training routine. So find that skirt you've been too shy to wear and show off your great new gams!

THIGHS AND CALVES
ULTRA-SHAPING THE LEGS

There's no doubt that leg exercises, especially squats, are very hard work. In fact thousands of women refuse to do any leg training at all. Yet all serious fitness women know that if they are to succeed, leg-training workouts must be executed with regularity.

Squats

The most all-encompasing leg exercise is the squat. It simply works the thighs in a more direct and intense fashion than any other exercise. Some argue that the leg press is actually an upside-down squat without the discomfort. While this exercise is a useful adjunct to the squat, it loses out in a direct comparison.

The back squat is definitely the muscle-growth exercise. Fully contoured upper legs cannot be built without squatting. If you are looking for more thigh size, then you must base your workout around the regular back squat. Squatting is a very natural exercise, but weight trainers did not use this movement extensively until the introduction of squat stands in the 1930s. Prior to that, lifters stood the barbell on end, hoisted it onto their shoulders, and then shuffled it into position across the back of their neck. It was all very time-consuming and dangerous. Thank heaven for squat stands! Unless you are a beginner, you should select at least two other quad movements and a leg-curl exercise in addition to squats.

The hack squat works the outer-thigh sweep and the lower part of the thighs near the knees. It has a thigh-lengthening effect.

Leg Extensions

The popular leg-extension exercise will not give you much development, but it has its use in that the quadriceps muscles are somewhat isolated and separated during the exercise. This, especially in conjunction with a clean nutrition program, will contribute to a sleeker quad appearance. Actually, if you lean back to the supine position, during this exercise you will notice that the muscles of the upper thighs, which run into the groin area, are also subjected to this muscle-isolating effect. (Note: Not all leg extension apparatus allow the torso to be tilted backwards.)

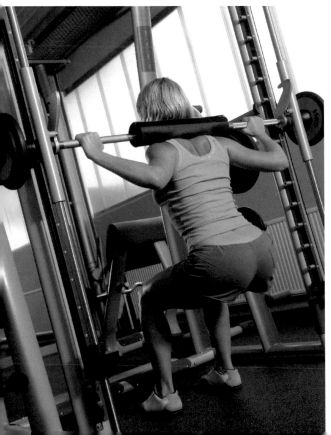

↖ Smith-machine squats

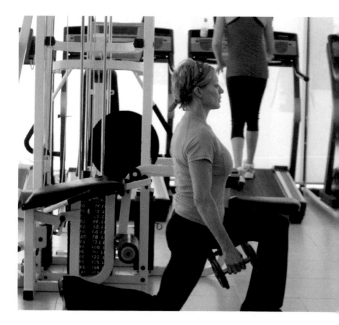

TIP

Don't let squats intimidate you! I have learned to love them.

Shape not Size

For those women who feel they have enough thigh muscle mass, it is probably wise to do *only* shaping exercises. In such a case, you may find it advantageous to use a Smith machine when performing deep-knee bends (squats). A Smith machine has a horizontal bar that can travel only upward or downward.

The advantage of Smith-machine squats is that you can alter your foot placement to put stress on different parts of the body. You can squat with your feet in front of the bar or behind it if you wish. This would be impossible using a free-weight barbell – you would fall over! Almost everyone should make sure the stress is on the middle and lower areas of the thigh. The farther forward your feet are placed the lower the area being worked. The regular back squat will build the upper thighs and glutes. Your job is to decide which is best for you, and keep to the selected style until results become evident.

Hamstrings

The leg biceps muscle at the back of the upper leg, also known as the hamstrings, is an extremely important muscle to develop. If you do not build up this area, the back of your leg will appear flat and lifeless. Leg curls work this area.

With a little ingenuity you can change the stress point to hit different parts of the leg biceps. For example, if the leg-curl machine were tilted to a 20- to 30-degree angle (head higher than legs), you would vigorously work the lower part of the biceps. A steeper angle (some leg-press machines even allow the exerciser to stand upright) will work the peak, or highest part of the hamstrings.

The usual method is to perform your leg curls on a relatively flat bench, with a slight rise in the middle to aid in lower-back protection. You can even involve your glutes, and tighten your butt while curling your legs. At the conclusion of the leg-curl movement try to lift your legs right off the bench. You can arch your back to maximize the effect. You'll need to use less weight for this variation.

THIG EXERCISES

SQUATS

Entire Thigh Area ▶▶▶▶

(8-20 REPS EACH SET)

Take a barbell from a pair of squat racks and hold it at the back of your neck. Roll a towel around the bar or use a special pad for added comfort. If needed, place your heels on a block of wood to improve your balance. Breathe in deeply before squatting. Keep your back flat and your head up throughout the movement. Breathe out forcefully as you rise up.

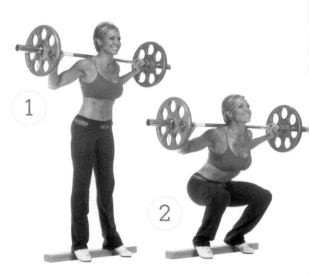

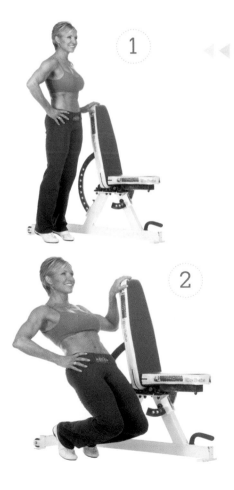

SISSY SQUATS

◀◀◀◀ Lower Thigh and General Sweep

(12-15 REPS EACH SET)

This specialized movement works the lower-thigh area. Use either no or very moderate weight. (Add weight by holding a barbell in front of the shoulders or by holding a dumbell at your side at arm's length.) The name "sissy squat" is not intended to denote that the exercise is easy. It is named after Sisyphus, who in Greek mythology was condemned to spend an eternity pushing a huge boulder up a mountain only to have it roll down again, forever to repeat the process.

The exercise is a little tricky. Adopt a position with your feet about 12 inches (30 cm) apart. Rise up on your toes and lower into a squat while leaning as far back as possible. Keep your thighs and torso in the same plane throughout the exercise. If this is too difficult, hold the back of a chair or sturdy upright structure for balance.

LUNGES

Thighs, Hips, Buttocks ▶ ▶ ▶ ▶

(10-20 REPS EACH SET)

Place a light barbell across your shoulders. Set your feet and legs comfortably apart. From the starting position, step forward two to three feet (60 to 90 cm) with your right leg. The longer the lunge the more it involves and firms the buttocks; the shorter the movement the more the thighs are stressed. When your right foot touches the floor, bend that leg as fully as possible. In the lunge position, your left knee should be about six to ten inches (15 to 25 cm) from the floor. Your torso will be arched and leaning slightly forward. Return to the original starting position and repeat the action with your left leg. Alternate the legs until the prescribed number of reps has been completed for both sides. Beginners should not use any resistance.

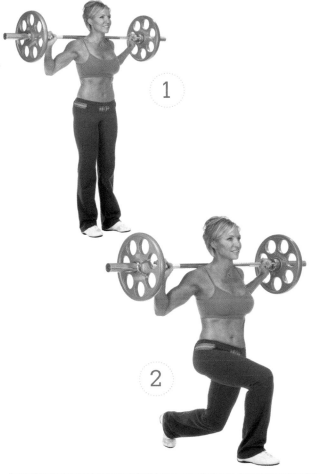

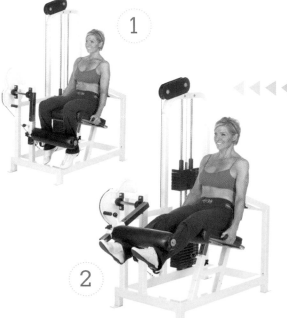

LEG EXTENSIONS

◀ ◀ ◀ ◀ Lower and Middle Thigh

(10-15 REPS EACH SET)

Sit on a leg-extension machine with your feet secured under the lift pad. Start lifting the weight by extending both legs together. Do not kick the weight up – start the lift slowly. If the machine you are using starts to move, you are exerting too much force. Slow down and make the muscles feel it rather than jerking the weight up.

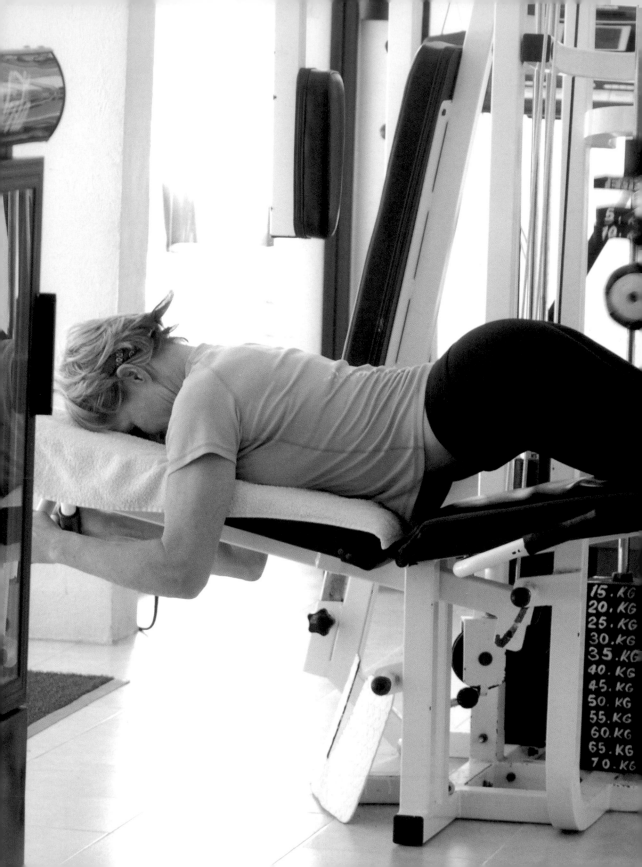

15.KG
20.KG
25.KG
30.KG
35.KG
40.KG
45.KG
50.KG
55.KG
60.KG
65.KG
70.KG

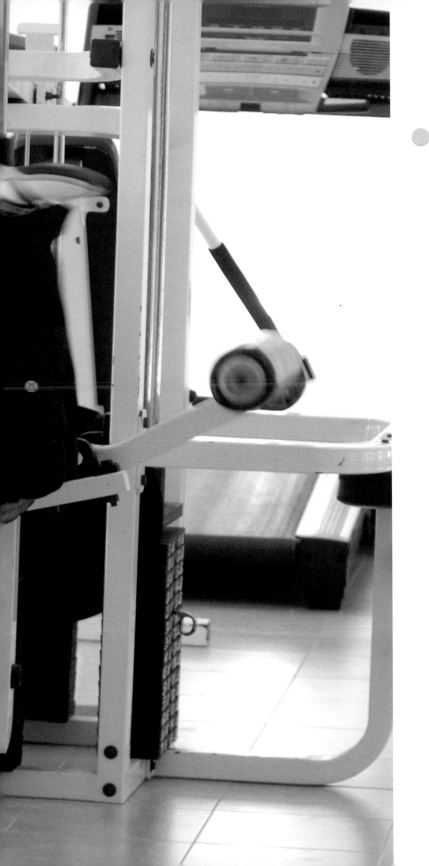

TIP

That wonderful burn in your "hams" after a leg workout is a sweet reminder you have done your best.

LEG CURLS

Thigh Biceps (Hamstrings) ▶ ▶ ▶ ▶

(12-15 REPS EACH SET)

Lie face down on a leg-curl machine. Hook your heels under the lift bar and curl your legs upward in unison. Concentrate on feeling the tension in the back of your legs. Do not bounce the weight up. Start each curl slowly and deliberately. You can prop your torso up on your elbows and lift your thighs to stress different areas. Some leg curl machines allow for an upright stance.

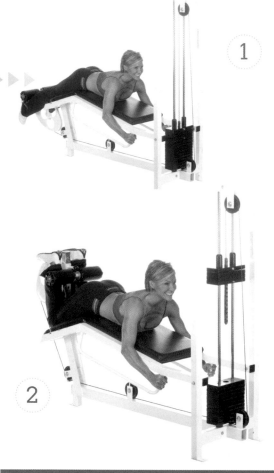

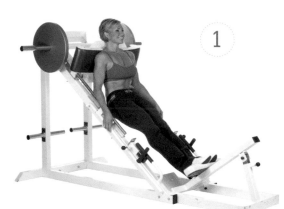

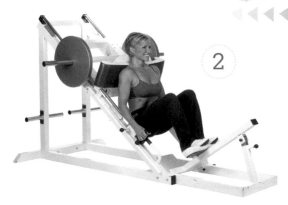

HACK SQUATS (HACK SLIDE)

◀ ◀ ◀ ◀ Middle and Lower Thigh

(10-15 REPS EACH SET)

Position yourself on a hack machine. Lower and lift yourself by bending and straightening your legs. You may find it advantageous to place your feet in a number of different positions (heels together with toes pointing outward will develop the outside of the thighs). Experiment by keeping your knees together and by taking a wider stance.

HACK LIFTS

Middle and Lower Thigh ▶▶▶▶

(10-15 REPS EACH SET)

Step in front of a loaded barbell. Reach back, grab hold and stand up. Hold your head up and squat down, keeping the bar close to the back of your legs as you do so. Rise and repeat. You can place a two-by-four-inch block of wood under your heels to help control your balance.

CALF EXERCISES

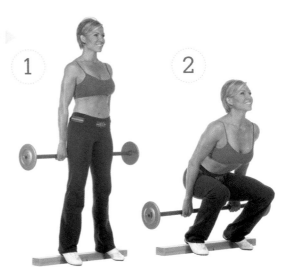

TIP

I put a lot of emphasis on stretching my calves to help them grow as much as possible.

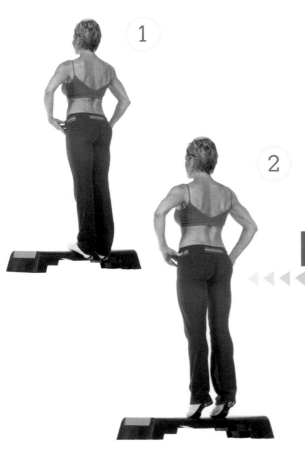

CALF RAISES

◀◀◀◀ Gastrocnemius

(15-25 REPS EACH SET)

When it comes to calf raises, make sure to go right up on your toes and get a good stretch at the bottom of the movement. Calves are endurance muscles and most people see the best results from higher reps.

SEATED CALF RAISES

Soleus ▶▶▶▶

(15-20 REPS EACH SET)

This exercise is performed on a special seated calf machine. The muscle worked in this movement is the one below the visible calf muscle. Perform as many heel raises as you can, concentrating on maximizing total calf stretch with each repetition. Make sure there is adequate padding on the T-hoist to fully protect your knees.

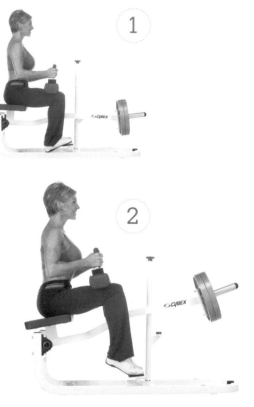

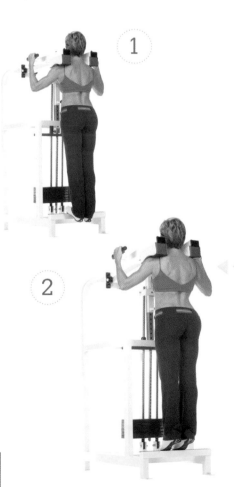

CALF-MACHINE RAISES

◀◀◀◀ Entire Calf

(15-25 REPS EACH SET)

The apparatus should be capable of giving you a great deal of resistance, as calves can take very heavy loads.

Keep your legs straight and go up and down on your toes as far as you can in both directions.

SINGLE-LEG CALF RAISES

Entire Calf ▶ ▶ ▶ ▶

(15-25 REPS EACH SET)

This exercise is very similar to the standing calf raise. You can do this exercise on a step or stair, holding a wall, standing on one foot and holding a dumbell, or you may do it on a calf machine. After a set with one leg, switch to the other.

TIP

Work with a partner if you find this equipment intimidating. You'll see it through together.

DONKEY CALF RAISES

◀ ◀ ◀ ◀ Gastrocnemius

(15-25 REPS EACH SET)

The bent-over position you adopt for donkey calf raises does something very special for the lower legs. Lean on a bench or table top so your upper body is comfortably supported and parallel to the floor. Have a training partner sit on your lower back, over the hip area – yes, really! Rise up and down on your toes until you cannot perform another rep. Use a step or block of wood for a greater range of motion. Some gyms have a donkey-calf machine. If yours does, make good use of it!

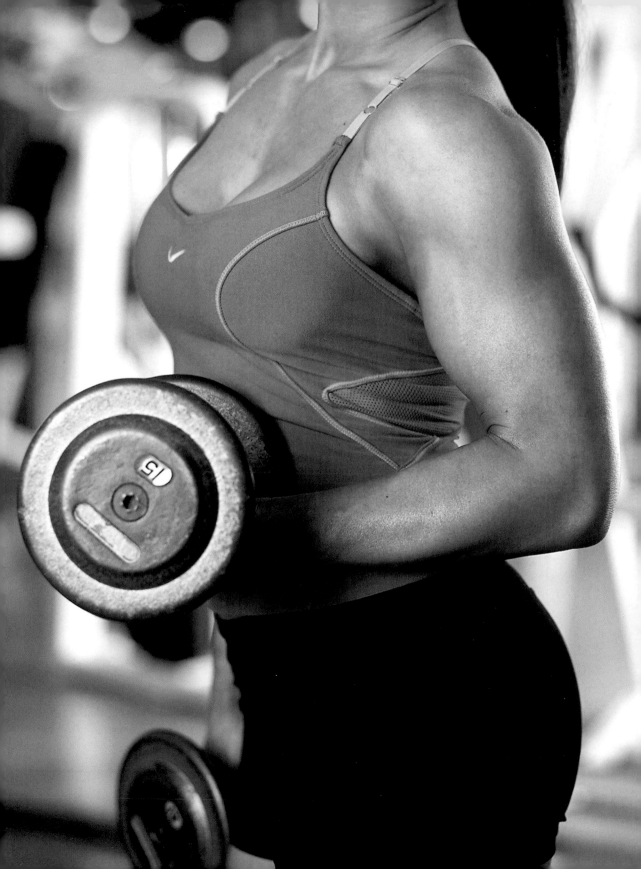

12

Lifting groceries and pushing the lawnmower will no longer be tiring tasks after you've added biceps and triceps exercises to your weight routine. Even better, tank tops will be wardrobe choice #1.

BICEPS & TRICEPS
SHAPING THE ARMS

Women today want to develop nicely muscled, balanced arms in the same way we strive for firm-looking legs and hips. No flabby wings for me please!

The arm is made up of the forearm muscles of the lower arm, and the triceps, brachialis, and biceps of the upper arm. The forearms are brought into action in every exercise you do. Whenever you pick up a barbell or dumbell, even for leg exercises, the forearm is activated. Like the calves, the forearms are endurance muscles and need higher reps.

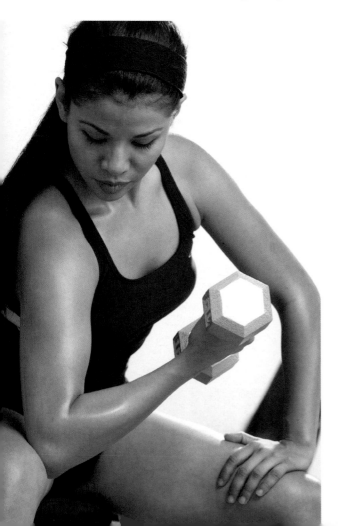

Biceps

When people say: "Show us your muscle!" they are invariably referring to the biceps. The biceps appear to be one long muscle that forms a bump when we bend our arm, but it is actually made up of two heads. The outer head of the biceps is exercised most when we perform close-grip curls or chins; the inside head is especially activated when we use a wide grip.

Triceps

The triceps have three distinct heads, which act to straighten the arms. Just as you should aim to build "low" biceps, it is also a good idea to try and build "low" triceps to give your arm proper shape. In my opinion, the most attractive triceps section is the outer head. This beautiful muscle is located just beneath the lateral deltoid (side shoulder). It is isolated in most triceps exercises where the elbows are held considerably wider than the hands.

Brachialis

The brachialis is not a particularly noticeable muscle in the upper arm, but its development is important if you want arm thickness. The brachialis develops from back exercises as well as curling exercises.

TIP

I am proud of having biceps and triceps definition in my arms. I wear short sleeves all the time!

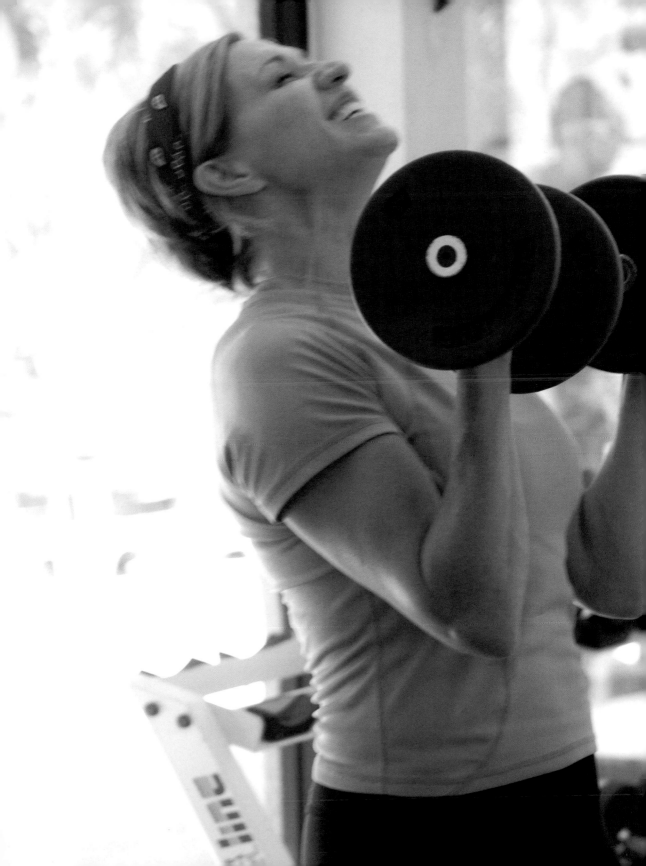

TRICEPS PRESSDOWNS

Entire Triceps ▶ ▶ ▶ ▶

(8-15 REPS EACH SET)

Hold a triceps bar with your hands two to eight inches (5 to 20 cm) apart. Press down until your arms are straight. Return to the start and repeat. Most people keep their elbows at their sides during this movement, but some deliberately hold the elbows out to the sides and lean into the exercise to activate the outer triceps head.

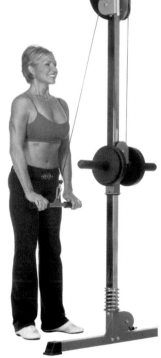

1

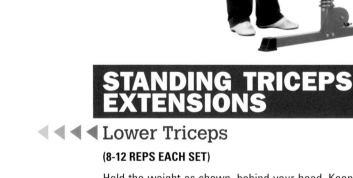

2

TIP

Once you get the hang of triceps training you will love the results.

1

2

STANDING TRICEPS EXTENSIONS

◀ ◀ ◀ ◀ Lower Triceps

(8-12 REPS EACH SET)

Hold the weight as shown, behind your head. Keep your elbows pointing skyward and as close to your head as possible. Lift and lower the weight rhythmically. Don't bounce at the bottom of the exercise, as this could strain the tendons near the elbow.

SINGLE-ARM LYING TRICEPS EXTENSIONS

Outside Triceps Head ▶ ▶ ▶ ▶

(12-15 REPS EACH SET)

Lie on your back on a flat exercise bench, your feet firmly on the floor. Hold a light dumbell in your right hand at arm's length above your chest. Keeping the upper arm as vertical as possible, bend your elbow until the dumbell touches your left shoulder. Lift steadily and repeat. Do not bounce the weight in this exercise. Perform the same movement with the left arm, lowering it to the right shoulder.

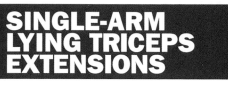

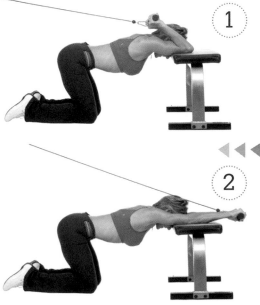

PRONE PULLEY TRICEPS EXTENSIONS

◀ ◀ ◀ ◀ Lower and Lateral Triceps

(10-15 REPS EACH SET)

Kneel on the floor, facing away from the cable stack and holding a pulley handle with both hands. Rest your elbows on a low bench. Slowly straighten your arms. Return to the start using control and repeat with a steady rhythm.

SINGLE-ARM DUMBELL EXTENSIONS

Lower Triceps ▶▶▶▶

(10-15 REPS EACH SET)

This triceps exercise develops the lower triceps area. Hold a dumbell above your head, and then lower it to the back of your neck, bending your arm at the elbow. Try to keep your upper arm close to your head. Avoid bouncing the weight at the bottom of the movement – doing so may cause elbow problems.

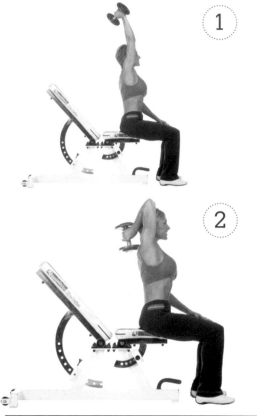

1

2

1

2

CLOSE-GRIP BENCH PRESSES

◀◀◀◀ Lateral Triceps Head

(6-10 REPS EACH SET)

Lie face up on a flat bench, feet firmly planted on the floor, holding a barbell (EZ-curl bars are the most popular) or have a partner hand it to you. Use a narrow grip so your hands are only 8 to 10 inches (20 to 25 cm) apart. Keeping your elbows close to your body, lower the weight to your breastbone and immediately push upwards. You should start by using only light weights.

LYING TRICEPS EXTENSIONS

Entire Triceps ▶▶▶▶

(8-12 REPS EACH SET)

Lie on your back as shown, and hold two dumbells at arms' length. Lower them slowly to your ears, and lift them again to the starting position. This exercise works the entire triceps area. Do not use heavy weights if you are prone to elbow or ligament soreness.

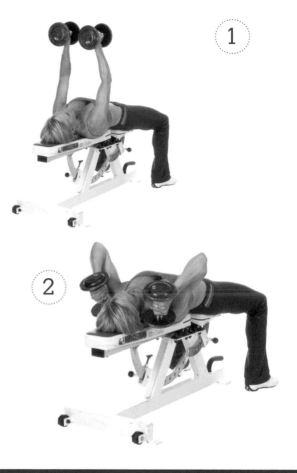

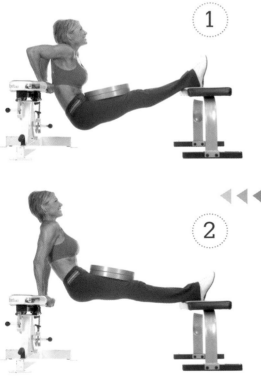

TRICEPS DIPS

◀◀◀◀ Triceps Belly

(10-20 REPS EACH SET)

Set yourself up as illustrated using benches or chairs and dip down as low as you can for each repetition. Press back up immediately until your arms are straight. If you are feeling strong, you may choose to place a weight disc on your upper thighs for added resistance. If this exercise is too difficult for you, place your feet on the floor.

BICEPS EXERCISES

BARBELL CURLS

Biceps Belly ▶▶▶▶

(6-12 REPS EACH SET)

Hold the bar slightly wider than shoulder width, and keep your elbows close to your body as you curl the weight upwards until it is under your chin.

There are two distinct styles of doing this exercise:

1) strictly (no leaning backwards during the movement, starting from a straight-arm position with absolutely no body motion or "swing"), and

2) cheating (hoisting the weight up by turning the trunk of your body into a pendulum as you swing the barbell). Both methods work. Most trainers get the best results by doing at least the first 6 to 8 reps in strict style and then finishing off the last more difficult 3 to 4 reps with a cheating motion.

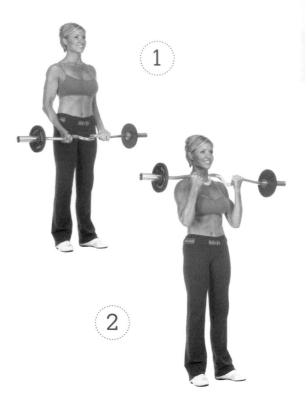

** Beautiful, powerful arms are the picture of feminine strength. Flex your biceps and show the world the wonder woman you are!

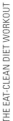

SEATED DUMBELL CURLS

Overall Biceps ▶ ▶ ▶ ▶

(8-12 REPS EACH SET)

Sit at the end of a flat bench, holding two dumbells. Curl them simultaneously to the shoulders and lower slowly. Try not to lean backwards as you curl the dumbells. Again, your palms may face either up or towards the body.

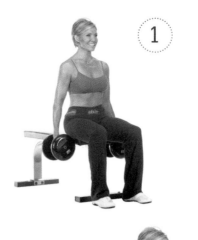

PULLEY CURLS

◀ ◀ ◀ ◀ Biceps Peak

(10-15 REPS EACH SET)

Hold a pulley cable handle (attached to a low pulley) with an underhand grip. Keeping your elbows close to the body, smoothly curl the bar up. You may have difficulty controlling the bar at first, but you will master the technique in no time.

ALTERNATE DUMBELL CURLS

Biceps Belly ▶▶▶▶

(6-10 REPS EACH SET)

This exercise is a great favorite of many champion bodybuilders. It works the biceps more directly than the two-handed dumbell curl, since it tends to prevent cheating.

Standing erect curl one dumbell. As you lower it, curl the other arm. Lower slowly, and do not swing the dumbells up with any added body motion.

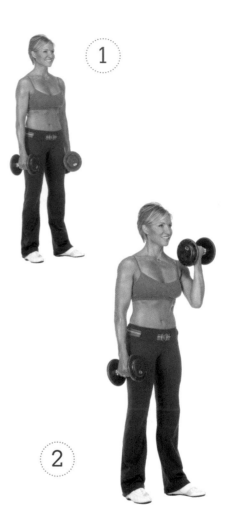

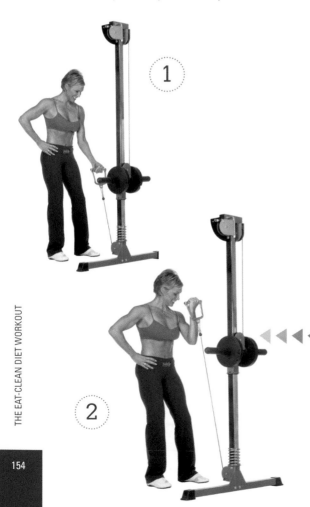

SINGLE-ARM PULLEY CURLS

◀◀◀◀ Biceps Peak

(10-15 REPS EACH SET)

Use the low pulley cable with the single-arm attachment. Start with the arms in a straight (extended) position and curl with a smooth, rhythmic action.

PREACHER-BENCH CURLS

Overall Biceps ▶▶▶▶

(8-12 REPS EACH SET)

Adopt a position with your arms over a preacher bench. Hold either a barbell (as shown) or a pair of dumbells. Curl up to the chin, and then lower slowly. Repeat. Do not bounce the weights when your arms are in the straight position. You can change the angle of most preacher benches to place the stress on different areas of the biceps. A 90-degree angle works the biceps peak, whereas a shallow 30-degree angle works the lower biceps. Perform this movement religiously and you will develop great biceps.

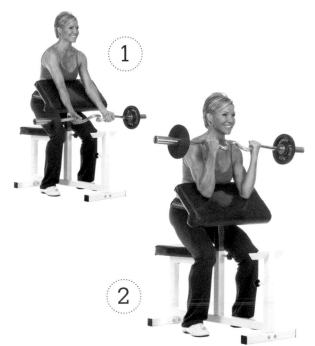

TIP

I love this exercise! Sometimes I get a better grip by standing rather than sitting.

STANDING DUMBELL CURLS

◀◀◀◀ Overall Biceps

(8-10 REPS EACH SET)

Adopt a comfortable standing position with your feet about 12 inches (30 cm) apart. Curl two dumbells simultaneously until they are next to your shoulders. Start with your palms facing your legs. While you lift the weights, turn your wrists until your palms are facing upwards. Lower the dumbells slowly and repeat.

PREACHER-BENCH WRIST CURLS

Forearm Flexors ▶▶▶▶

(10-15 REPS EACH SET)

Adopt a position with your arms over a preacher bench as shown, restricting the movement to the wrists. Curl the hands in a deliberate and forceful manner. Concentrate the action of the exercise into your lower arms.

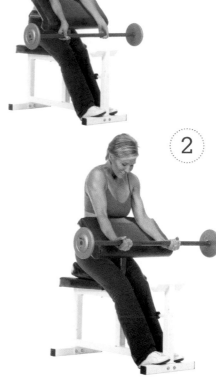

1

2

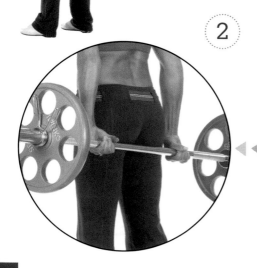

1

2

BEHIND-BACK WRIST CURLS

◀◀◀◀ Forearm Flexors

(12-15 REPS EACH SET)

Standing, hold a barbell behind your back with an under-hand grip. Lift the hands rearwards and upwards. Restrict all movements to the hands and wrists only.

REVERSE CURLS

Forearm Extensors ▶▶▶▶

(12-15 REPS EACH SET)

Stand erect, holding a barbell slightly wider than shoulder width. Hold a barbell at arms' length with your palms facing back. This is called a reverse grip. Curl the barbell, keeping your wrists straight and your elbows tucked in. Lower and repeat. You will feel this exercise in the upper forearm, near the elbow. Use considerably less weight in this exercise than for the regular barbell curl.

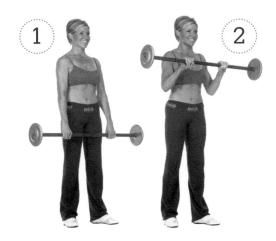

WRIST CURLS

◀◀◀◀ Forearm Belly

(12-15 REPS EACH SET)

Wrist curls work the flexors (the belly) of the forearm. Sit with your lower arms resting on your knees or on the top of a padded bench. Hold the dumbells with both hands with your palms facing up. Moving only your wrists, curl the weight up until your forearms are fully contracted. Allow the dumbells to lower under control.

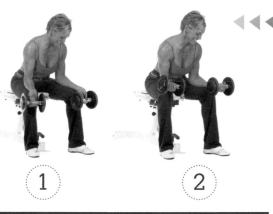

REVERSE WRIST CURLS

Forearm Extensors ▶▶▶▶

(12-15 REPS EACH SET)

Kneel at a flat bench with one arm across the bench. Hold a dumbell in one hand with an overhand grip. This is called a reverse grip. Rest the other hand on your working forearm. Curl the dumbell, moving your wrists only. Lower the dumbell with control.

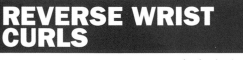

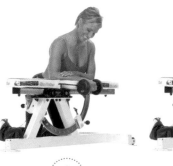

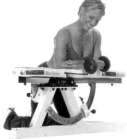

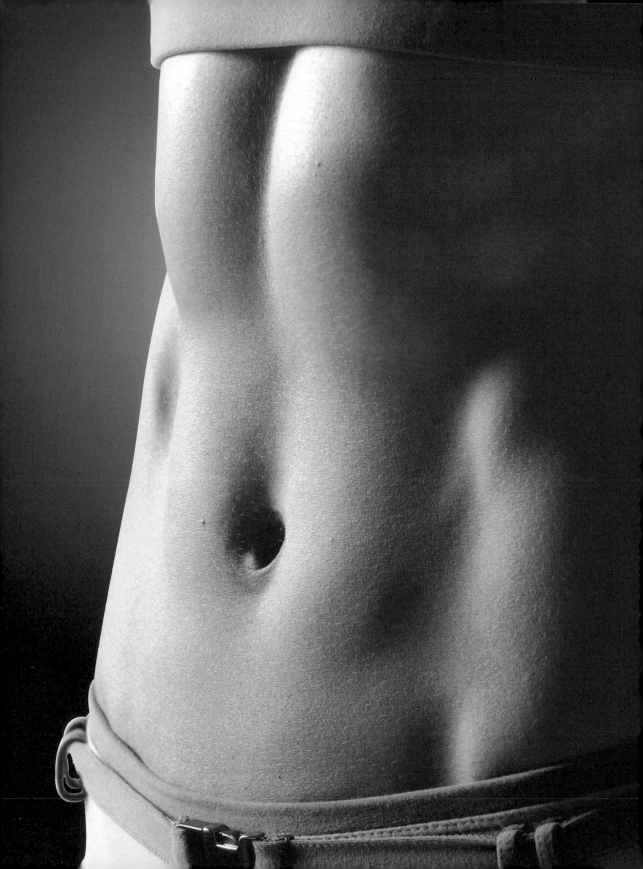

13

Let's face it, everyone wants great abs! Whether you're after a defined midsection or a sweet six-pack, it's possible by doing a few of my favorite exercises. Be bikini worthy once and for all!

WAIST REDUCTION
SHAPING YOUR ABS

As with any muscle group, the abdominals are developed with progressive-resistance exercise. And like any other area, they are defined by keeping a focused habit of Eating Clean and avoiding calorie-dense junk foods.

So many people think they will get lean, nicely defined abs by doing crunches and leg raises, and this is simply not the case. There is little direct link between abdominal exercises and fat reduction around the waist area. A three-mile walk will do more to help your waistline than several sets of ab exercises because the walk burns more fuel. Top fitness women know that abdominals are *built* with quality waist exercise and *honed* with diet and aerobic activity. Want your abs to show? Then you have to make a habit of Eating Clean.

Some women have stomach muscles with straight, lined-up ridges, while others appear to have more uneven abs. This is genetically predetermined, and cannot change. An uneven ab formation should never count against you in competition. A well-conditioned waistline is what counts the most.

Some experts, such as trainer-to-the-stars Gunnar Peterson and other noted experts, decree that the abdominals require no more than 15 to 12 repetitions for maximum growth and tone, and that more repetitions are only a waste of time. Other experts, such as Elaine Goodlad and Mindi O'Brien, feel that very high-repetition movements are more advantageous.

TIP

For me, the biggest change in my waist size came from combining Clean Eating with abdominal training. That's when the results arrived!

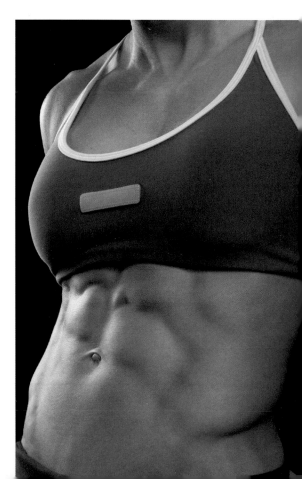

Both methods work. The question is whether high repetitions are actually more effective than low reps. I think the best recommendation is to train using the method that suits your personality. If you feel more comfortable using less resistance with 100 or 200 reps per set, then carry on. Or perhaps you prefer to add resistance and do 10 to 15 reps. Pros like Monica Brant like to use 15 to 30 reps in most of their ab training, whereas I stay around 35 reps.

If you haven't been doing many waist exercises lately, don't make the mistake of suddenly throwing yourself into a hectic ab workout. The midsection forms the nerve center of the body, and too much ab work too soon can throw your bodily functions for a loop. Ease your way into any new abdominal-training program if you want maximum results.

For clear-cut, sharp abdominal muscles, you must think either in terms of diet or of physically burning up more calories each day. The best and fastest method is to attack the problem on both fronts. Eat a Clean diet *and* increase your cardio workouts, and your slender waist will appear!

Two additional tips: Never push your stomach out (even for a joke): this can overstretch the abdominal wall, never to return to normal. You can liken the effect to a spring that is pulled out to a point beyond which it will spring back – the strain in the metal has caused a rupture and nothing will induce it to regain its elasticity. The wearing of a weightlifting belt during your workouts will help prevent "overstretch." Another tip is to avoid taking any type of thyroid, steroid or human growth hormone drug, because each can lead to a bloated waistline area as a disastrous side effect.

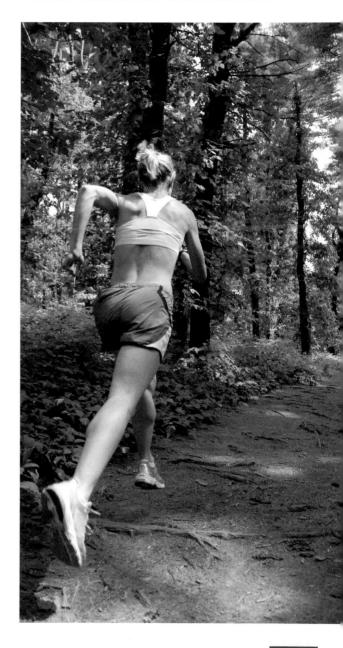

PARTIAL CRUNCHES

Entire Abdomen ▶▶▶▶

(8-15 REPS EACH SET)

Lie on the floor or mat with your knees raised. You may cross your ankles, hold your feet together or hold them apart. Attempt to lift your shoulders from the floor while drawing your knees toward your face. Lower your shoulders and legs simultaneously.

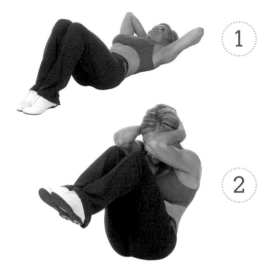

1

2

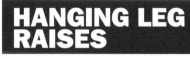

1

2

HANGING LEG RAISES

◀◀◀◀ Lower Abdominals

(12-25 REPS EACH SET)

Hang from an overhead horizontal bar, with your arms about 20 inches (50 cm) apart. Keep your legs straight and lift them until they are just past the parallel-to-floor position. Lower and repeat. Try not to let your body build up a swinging motion.

If you are unable to perform this exercise with straight legs, start off with your knees bent. Tuck your knees into your waist with each repetition, and point your toes downward. Start slowly, with no swinging. After a few weeks you should be able to graduate to the straight-leg style.

THE EAT-CLEAN DIET WORKOUT

SEATED BENT-KNEE TUCKS

Entire Abdomen ▶ ▶ ▶ ▶

(15-20 REPS EACH SET)

Adopt a position on a flat exercise bench as shown. Hold the bench to fix your body at the correct angle. Lift your knees up to your chest and then straighten. Keep the stress on the waist area by holding your torso position until the end of the exercise.

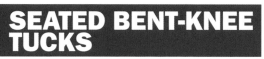

SIDE TWISTS

◀ ◀ ◀ ◀ Obliques and Intercostals

(50-300 REPS EACH SET)

Not all fitness followers believe in the effectiveness of this exercise. It does, however, mobilize the waist area, and the oblique muscles are worked quite strongly despite little or no resistance. Your flexibility will also improve. As you twist from side to side, make a conscious effort to keep your hips facing forward.

SIDE BENDS

Obliques ▶▶▶▶

(15 + REPS EACH SET)

Stand in the upright position, feet comfortably apart, toes pointing slightly outward. Bend with a forceful effort, first to one side and then the other. When your body gets used to this movement you may hold a dumbell in one hand. After the allocated number of repetitions, hold the dumbell in the other hand and repeat.

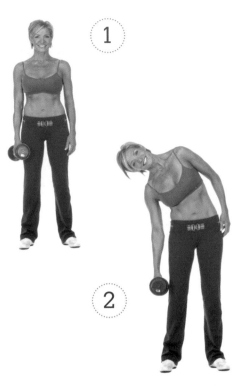

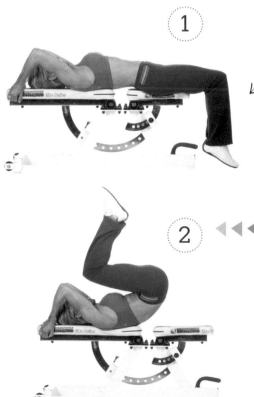

↖ *This is my all-time favorite ab exercise. Talk about a challenge!*

REVERSE CRUNCHES

◀◀◀◀ Lower and Middle Abdominals

(15-30 REPS)

Lie on your back on a flat bench. Clasp your hands behind your head at the sides of the bench. Keeping your knees bent throughout, lift your legs with control from the floor and back until your butt lifts off the bench. Lower till your toes just kiss the floor.

BENCH CRUNCHES

Middle and Upper ▶▶▶▶ Abdominals

(10-15 REPS EACH SET)

Lie on your back on the floor. Rest your calves on a bench so your thighs are vertical. Place your hands behind your head and slowly attempt to sit up. This movement is far more effective than a regular sit-up, because tension is kept constant in the middle and upper abdominals.

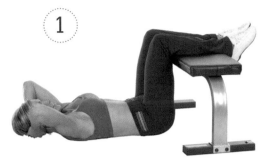

1

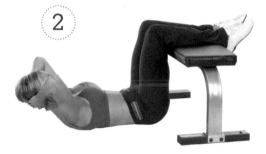

2

1

2

BENT-OVER TWISTS

◀◀◀◀ Side and Intercostal Areas

(30 + REPS EACH SET)

Start by getting into position shown. Hold a bar or a broomstick behind your head, against your shoulders. Twist deliberately to both sides while holding your base position.

CAPTAIN'S CHAIR KNEE RAISES

Upper, Mid and Lower ▶▶▶▶ Abdominals

(15-30 REPETITIONS EACH SET)

Position yourself in the Captain's chair with your back firmly against the back support and forearms on the arm rests. Your legs should be hanging freely. Contract your abs to bring your knees up toward your chest. Relax your legs, letting them hang again. Repeat. Do not swing your legs. Use control to lift and lower them to directly challenge the abs.

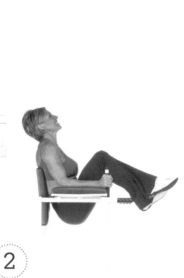

1

2

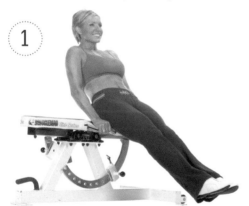

1

2

JACKKNIVES

◀◀◀◀ Mid and Lower Abdominals

(15-30 REPETITIONS EACH SET)

Sit on the side edge of a flat bench with your hands on either side of you for support. Lean back slightly. Place your feet straight out in front of you on the floor. Keeping your legs straight, lift them as high as you can. Lower to the starting position and repeat.

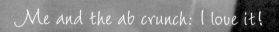
Me and the ab crunch: I love it!

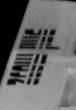

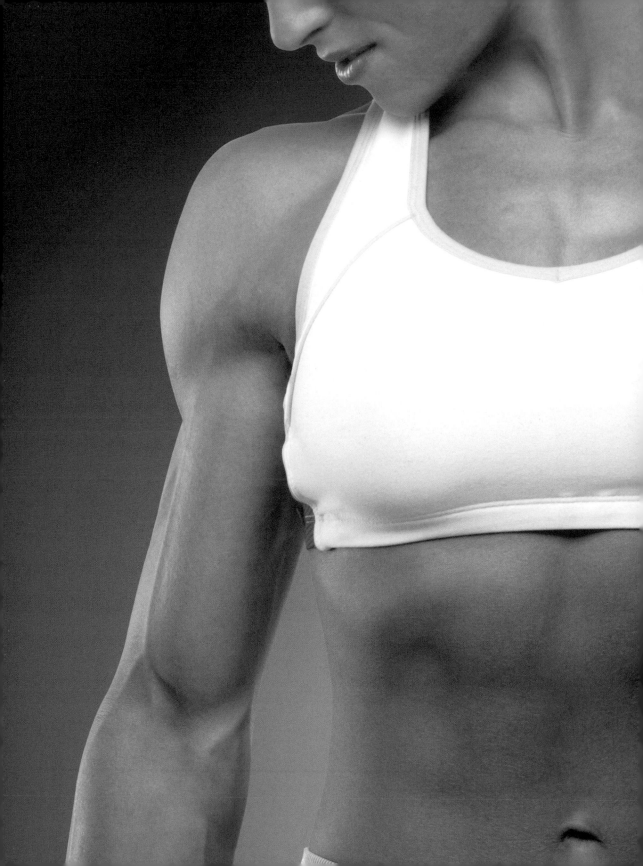

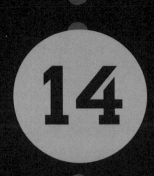

14

Throw out your shoulder pads! They are so 1984. Deltoid exercises are the best way to give your upper body some oomph. Even better, your new muscle tone will remain long after you take off your jacket.

SHOULDER SHAPING
CREATING DELIGHTFUL DELTS

Shoulder width and deltoid size used to be the exclusive domain of men. Until as recently as 20 years ago a woman wanted a neck that sloped delicately into her arms, with no shoulders to speak of. Today women want well-developed delts and squared-off shoulders that announce strength *and* look great in strapless dresses! The deltoid is a three-headed muscle positioned at the end of your collarbone. Its three distinct functions are to raise the arm forward, sideways, and backwards.

You need to work your shoulders from different angles to bring about complete-looking development, but be careful. Deltoids are easily overtrained and injuries can occur. Without proper rest and good exercise form, you could sustain ligament, tendon, or even rotator cuff injuries.

If you are lucky enough to have naturally wide shoulders, you should need little deltoid specialization. Women with narrow shoulders, however, must work very hard, building the delts from every angle, especially the lateral (side) head, which gives the most width to the body.

Make sure to warm up each deltoid head as you start working it, even if you have been using it as a secondary muscle: for example, doing bench presses. When attacking a complicated area such as the deltoids (with its three distinct heads) always begin each different movement with a light warm-up weight. This allows the fibers and tendons time to adjust to the new direction of stress.

DUMBELL PRESSES
Front and Side Shoulders
(8-10 REPS EACH SET)

Stand or sit, holding two dumbells at your shoulders. Keep your back straight and your head up. Press both dumbells simultaneously to the overhead position. Do not lean backwards during the exercise. Lower and repeat with a steady rhythm.

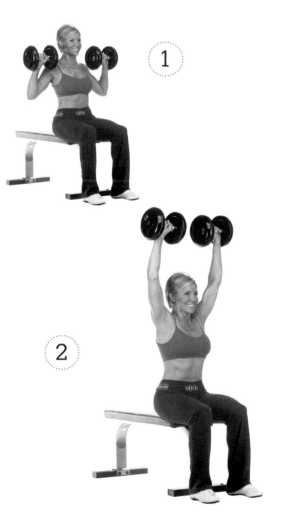

LATERAL RAISES

◀◀◀◀ Side Deltoids

(8-12 REPS EACH SET)

There are dozens of ways to perform this exercise, all with one purpose – to work the side deltoids. You can stand or sit, feet together or apart. However, to throw stress where you want it – on the lateral deltoids – you must bend your arms almost at right angles. Lift the weights to level with your head, and immediately lower. Keep your palms facing downwards throughout. At the time of peak effort, try to lean a little forward rather than back.

UPRIGHT ROWS

Deltoids and Traps ▶▶▶▶

(8-15 REPS EACH SET)

A narrow grip will work the frontal deltoids and the trapezius. A wider grip will put more stress on the side deltoids. Always straighten the arms at the bottom of the exercise and start your pull slowly, gathering momentum as the weight rises to your sternum. Keep the up-down movement rhythmic. Maintain an upright stance with feet comfortably apart. As the bar rises, try to keep your elbows as high as possible, and do not lean backwards.

INCLINE REAR LATERALS

Rear Deltoids ▶▶▶▶

(12-15 REPS EACH SET)

Sit backwards (facing the rear) on an incline bench, set at about a 35- to 40-degree angle. Lift and lower two light dumbells, tilting them slightly forward as if you were pouring from a pitcher. Your arms should be unlocked at the elbows rather than straight, to alleviate pressure. Do not swing your arms upwards. Start slowly and force the rear deltoids to lift the weight. Put your mind into the muscle.

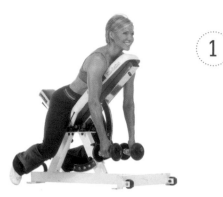

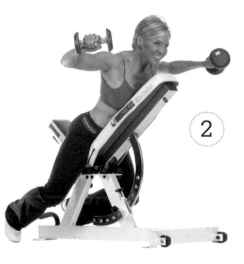

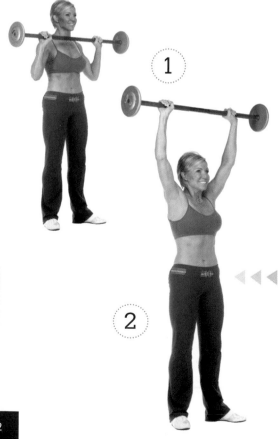

STANDING BARBELL PRESSES

◀◀◀◀ Front and Side Shoulders

(8-12 REPS EACH SET)

Stand with your feet comfortably apart. Holding the barbell at your shoulders, press the weight straight up, being careful not to lean too far back. Lock your arms briefly at the top of the movement. Lower and repeat.

PRESSES BEHIND NECK

Side Deltoids ▶▶▶▶

(6-12 REPS EACH SET)

Sit at a bench with back support. Hold a loaded barbell above your head with your hands spaced moderately far apart. (Your forearms should be approximately vertical.) Lower the weight behind your neck as far as possible. Lift it immediately. Do not bounce the bar from your shoulders. Keep your elbows as far back as possible throughout the movement. Press upwards and downwards in a complete repetition rhythmically, without pause. Do not do this exercise if your shoulders are stiff or if you feel pain.

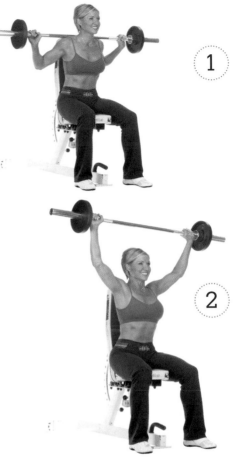

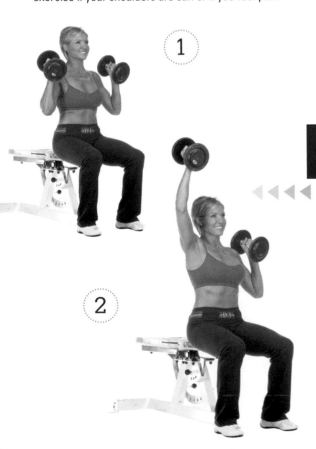

ALTERNATING DUMBELL PRESSES

◀◀◀◀ Side Deltoids

(8-12 REPS EACH SET)

Sit on a flat bench holding a pair of dumbells at your shoulders, palms facing inward or forward. Hold elbows back to maintain stress on your side deltoids. Start with your weakest hand, and alternately press first one dumbell and then the other in a seesaw fashion, with complete reps. Lower and continue the exercise with no pauses until the end of the set.

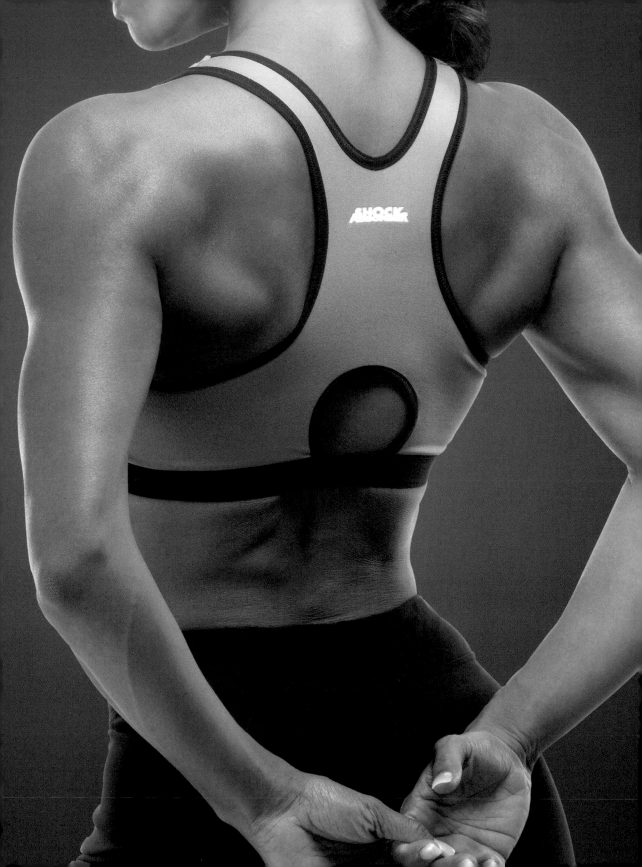

15

An hourglass figure is not just for that classic 1950's pin-up girl. Weight training is the best way to build up a little here and slim down a little there. Corsets need not apply!

BACK BEAUTY
THE HOURGLASS FIGURE

Throughout history the hourglass figure has been thought of as the epitome of beauty in a woman's physique. In the past we used corsets to accomplish this; now we use weights. Nothing does more to develop that shape than a wide upper back tapering to a tiny waist.

Since virtually all bodybuilders (male and female) renowned for their wide and dramatic V-shaped backs use wide-grip chins and pulldowns in their training, I suggest that a wide grip works better than a narrow or medium grip, although there is some argument about this. Perhaps you would like to experiment for yourself, but keep in mind that a narrow grip permits more biceps help, so your back will not be worked as fully.

All back exercises work the entire back, but different exercises put the stress on different areas. Put simply, the width of the back (the flair, or the V-shape) is built with pulldowns and chins, the thickness of the back is created mostly from rows, and hyperextensions are responsible for lower-back development. The trapezius, the muscle between the neck and the shoulders, is normally considered a back muscle, because it covers most of the middle part of the upper back. It is worked with shrug exercises and all rowing and pulley motions.

TIP
Now that I have worked hard on training my back, my V-taper is better and my waist looks smaller.

> **"Nothing does more to develop that shape than a wide upper back tapering to a tiny waist."**

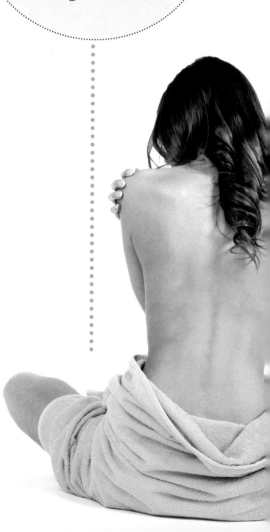

BENT-OVER BARBELL ROWS

Lower Lats ▶ ▶ ▶ ▶

(8-12 REPS EACH SET)

This exercise works the belly of the latissimus dorsi. Being careful not to round your back, bend and grasp a barbell from the floor. Keeping your head up and back straight, lift and lower the barbell to your abdomen. (To make sure your back is straight, push your rear out — it feels silly at first, but it works!)

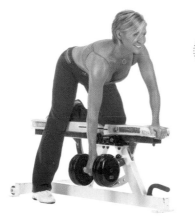

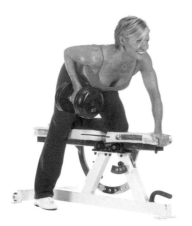

SINGLE-ARM DUMBELL ROWS

◀ ◀ ◀ ◀ Middle Lats

(8-12 REPS EACH SET)

Another total lat exercise, but one that eliminates lower-back strain, since your free arm is used to support your upper body. With control and no yanking, pull the dumbell up into the midsection, and lower until your arm is extended all the way down ... then try to lower it even more. Maximize the stretch.

INCLINE DUMBELL ROWS

Overall Lat and Upper Back ▶ ▶ ▶ ▶

(8-12 REPS EACH SET)

Sit backwards on an incline bench. Holding a dumbell in each hand, pull upwards with a strong rowing motion. Lower slowly until your arms are completely straight in the "down" position. Lift and lower with an even rhythm.

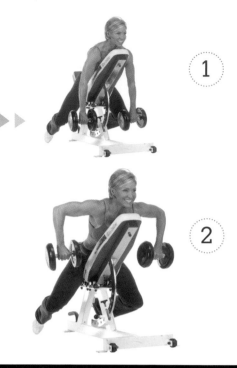

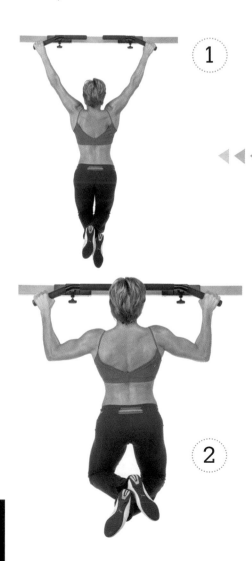

WIDE-GRIP CHINS

◀ ◀ ◀ ◀ Lat Width

(8-15 REPS EACH SET)

Grasp an overhead bar using an overhand grip at least a foot wider than your shoulders on either side. Pull yourself up, keeping your elbows back throughout the movement. You can bring yourself up to the front or the back of the bar. Lower until your arms are straight and repeat. (Note: Most women will have difficulty performing even one chin when they start exercising, especially if they are overweight. If this is the case for you, you can use a machine called an "assisted chin/dip machine." Anyone who works at your gym should be able to show you how to use it. If you do not have access to one of these machines, then use a chair or bench to take part of your weight while you pull yourself up.)

NARROW UNDER-GRIP CHINS

Lower Lats ▶▶▶▶

(8-15 REPS EACH SET)

Grab a standard overhead chinning bar with a fairly close grip, palms facing the body. Start by hanging with straight arms. Begin the pullup or chin with a slow, concentrated effort. Do not jerk or jump up from the floor. Rise until your chin is above the level of the bar; lower under control and repeat. (See Note regarding wide-grip chins, page 178.)

Don't get frustrated if you can do only one chin. Start there and work your way up! It will happen.

PARALLEL-GRIP CHINS

◀◀◀◀ Lat Belly

(10-15 REPS EACH SET)

Some chinning bars have parallel grips. If yours does not, you can hook a parallel handle over top as shown in this picture. Grap hold of the handles, hang straight down and then pull yourself up until your chin reaches just over your hands. Let yourself back down slowly. If this is too difficult for you, use a lat machine with a handle that allows your hands a parallel position. Keeping your back straight throughout the movement, pull the handle towards your upper chest. Slowly allow the bar back up under control and repeat.

LAT-MACHINE PULLDOWNS

V-Shape Development ▶▶▶▶

(10-15 REPS EACH SET)

Take a wide overhand grip on the bar, and pull down as far as you can. This exercise is not as effective as the wide-grip chinning exercise, but it does have these advantages: you can use less resistance if necessary, and you can pull the bar lower, working your lats over a greater range of motion.

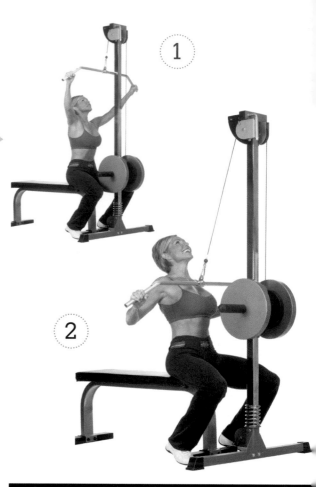

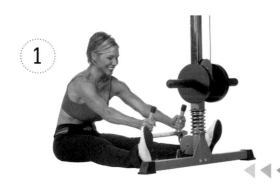

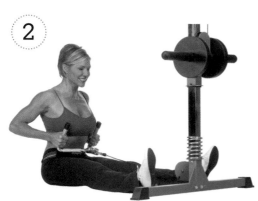

SEATED ROW

◀◀◀◀ Middle Back

(10-15 REPS EACH SET)

Attach a V-bar to a pulley on its lowest setting. Sit on the floor or machine's seat with feet out in front of you and a slight bend in your knees. Reach forward with a flat back and grab the bar with both hands. Pull the bar into your midsection as you bring your back to a straight position. Focus on squeezing your elbows together as much as possible. Make good use of the seated row machine at your local gym.

DEAD LIFTS

Lower and Overall Back ▶ ▶ ▶ ▶

(5-10 REPS EACH SET)

Bend over a loaded barbell with your feet comfortably apart. Grip the barbell with one hand under and the other hand over the bar, hands about shoulder-width apart. Straighten your back, bend your knees, and pull the bar up as you straighten to a standing position. Keep your head up throughout the exercise. Lower and repeat. Do not bounce the weight on the floor.

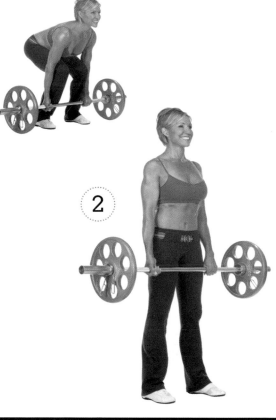

1

2

PRONE HYPEREXTENSIONS

◀ ◀ ◀ ◀ Lower Back

(10-20 REPS EACH SET)

This is performed on an exercise unit especially designed for the job. Climb into the unit and hold your body in a straight line. Your upper body should be free to bend up and down. Hold your hands behind your head. Bend at the hips, then straighten. You may eventually choose to hold a weight disc at your chest during this exercise.

GOOD-MORNING EXERCISE

▼ ## Lower Back

▼ **(10-15 REPS EACH SET)**

▼ Stand with your legs comfortably apart, a barbell across your shoulders. Keep your back straight. Rounding will injure your lower back. Bend forward at the hips and straighten up. Hold your head as high as you can throughout the movement. You may want to wrap a towel around the bar to prevent chafing at the neck. Your knees should be very slightly bent throughout. If your lower back is weak you will want to strengthen it with hyperextensions before moving on to good mornings. Use a light weight to start.

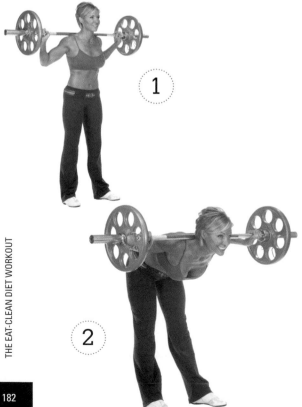

TIP

Training the back is rewarding because it responds quickly, and a carved back looks amazing in low-cut clothes or a swimsuit.

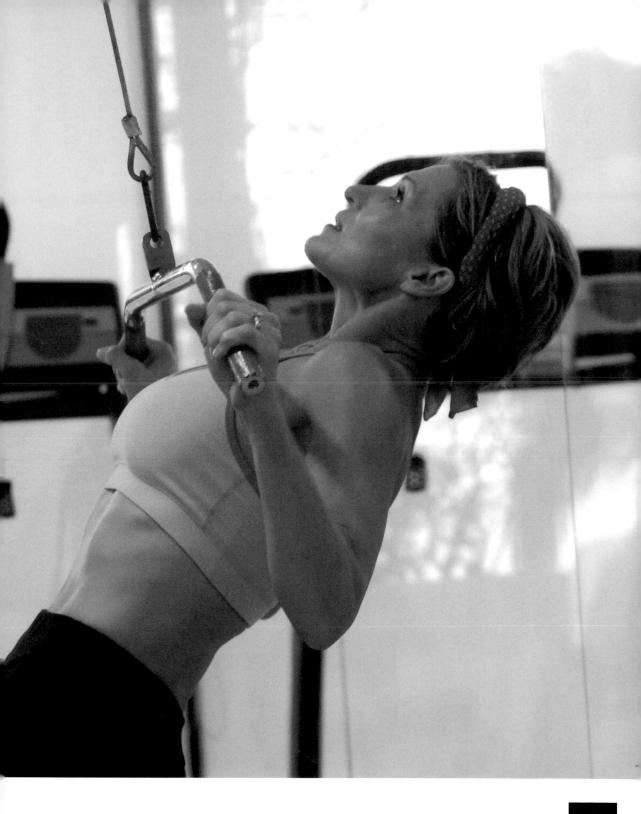

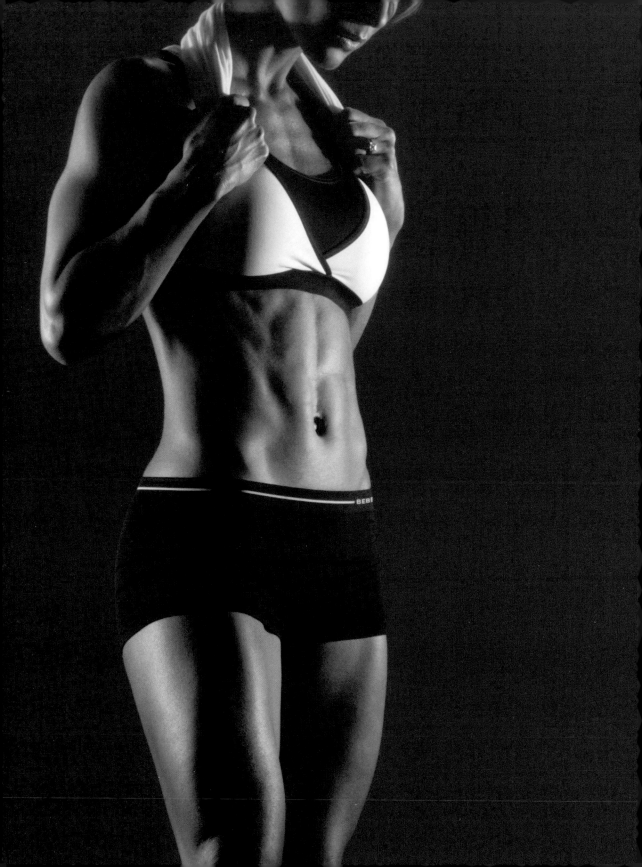

16

From straight sets to supersets, weight training has become its own field of study and it's easy to get overwhelmed! Use this chapter to clear up any confusion and personalize your workouts even more.

TRAINING PRINCIPLES
A SCIENTIFIC ART

Body sculpting is not just weight lifting. It is now a scientific practice involving many complex principles and theories. Today this art is quite sophisticated, and as time goes on and the body's feedback mechanisms are more identifiable and transferable to computer language, the scientific component of body shaping will grow even larger.

Bodybuilders have been using their own training "secrets" for scores of years, each method refined from preceding ones. Almost every book or magazine publisher has brought out a different system.

The first modern weight trainer, Eugen Sandow, introduced his dumbell training system in the late 1800s. He sold a light pair of dumbells with his training course. He was followed by Charles Atlas, with his own non-apparatus course. Then came Earle Leiderman, George Jowett, Peary Rader, Bob Hoffman, Joe Weider and Robert Kennedy. Out of all the experimentation and empirical evaluation a scientific system evolved. Today we have scores of weight-training principles – some of dubious distinction, which I have left out of this chapter. Others have a very definite place and should be explained.

I don't want to confuse you with too many routines and principles, but as you progress you will want to change up your routine every few weeks. Why? Because variety is the spice of progress. The body adapts to progressive resistance training. Once it gets used to a routine, it stops improving. When we surprise our muscles on a regular basis we maximize our muscle tone, metabolism and fat loss. We end up fitter, healthier and looking fabulous! Together we'll discover a few of the more popular and workable systems.

Straight Sets

The straight-set system is used by more weight trainers than any other method. "Straight sets" simply means that the trainer performs a set of a particular exercise, rests for 30 to 90 seconds, and then resumes with additional sets of the same exercise, allowing for a rest after each set. The trainer groups the exercises for each body part together, rather than doing, say, one exercise for chest, then doing squats, then doing another exercise for chest. Virtually every weight trainer has used this straight-set system more than any other.

Heavy-Duty Training

This technique pushes the body's capacity until the muscle being exercised actually fails in the completion of a repetition. Heavy-duty training is the logical way to train when one considers that scientific data proves a muscle grows only when it is subjected to an ever-increasing workload.

The key word for this technique is intensity, which requires excessive effort on behalf of the trainer. Because of the high degree of effort required in a heavy-duty set, a typical heavy-duty program contains only one or two sets per exercise, not including a warm-up set. Heavy-duty training is not for beginners or intermediates. It is an advanced technique.

This is one of my favorite ways to train!

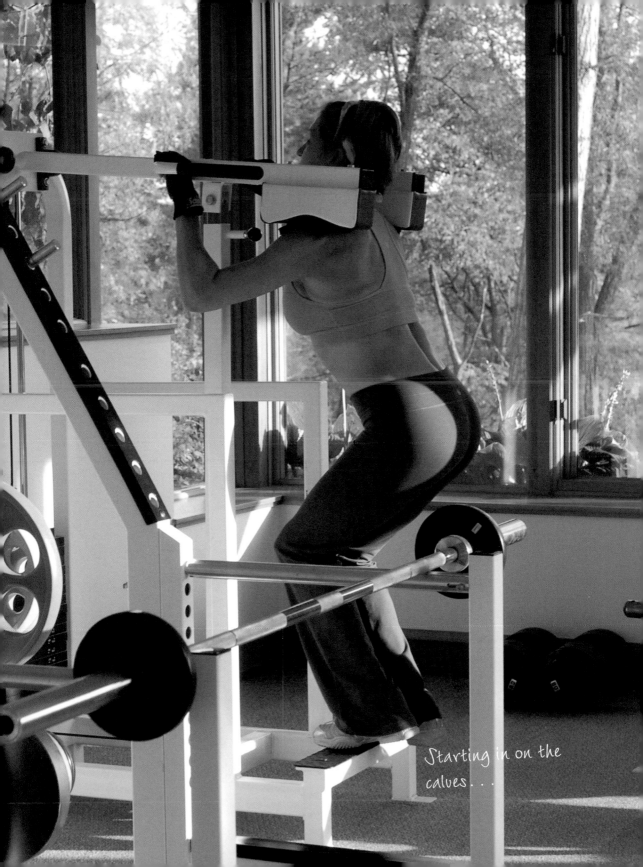

Starting in on the calves...

Supersets

All muscles contract and shorten. When this occurs, the tendon attached to the muscle then pulls on a bone, moving that part of the anatomy. The biceps muscle contracts and pulls the forearm upwards. The triceps muscle, in back of the arm, pulls the forearm back down. Weight trainers, however, call them pulling and pushing muscles. Pushing exercises include standing shoulder presses, supine bench presses, push-ups, triceps extensions and leg presses. Pulling exercises refer to upright rows, curls, chins, bent-over rows and leg curls.

The original idea of supersets was to alternate two exercises for opposing muscles, rapidly and without rest – one pulling and one pushing movement. For example, one could alternate biceps curls with triceps extensions. Many trainers simply alternate two curling movements, two pectoral movements or two triceps movements, not caring whether a particular muscle was being worked against another (for example, the biceps and triceps). Today, supersets merely refer to the alternation of any two exercises in rapid succession.

This type of exercise can jolt the muscles into new tone in weeks, but it is very severe. Too many supersets could cause you to become overtrained, bringing your progress to a standstill. Paradoxically, you can break a standstill with a week or two of supersetting your exercises.

If a training partner helps you lift the weight, you can still lower it yourself. This is called a "negative."

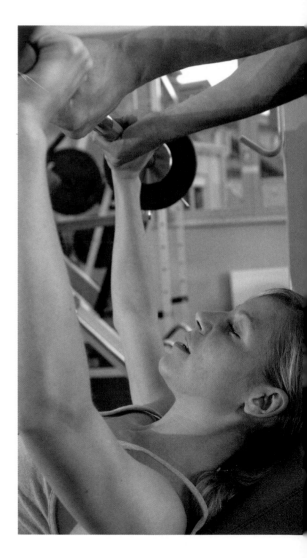

Forced Negatives and Forced Reps

The lifting of a weight is known as concentric contraction, while the lowering of a weight (returning to starting position from the point of full contraction) is known as eccentric contraction. When you cannot perform another repetition of an exercise you can call upon a training partner to assist by giving a light touch to the bar as you lift it. This is known as a "forced rep," because without the help you could not successfully complete the exercise. Once you can no longer complete a concentric contraction you can still manage a few eccentric contractions. If a training partner helps you lift the weight, you can still lower it yourself. This is called a "negative."

Let's imagine you are performing a standing barbell curl. You manage eight good reps on your own (unassisted). Normally you would end the set there. However, you can further stress the muscle by having a training partner stand in front of you and use a finger to give you just enough help to get the weight up while you perform yet another curl (forced rep). Then you can compound the effect even more by lowering the weight slowly (negative rep).

Negative reps are not suitable for everyone. You have to have an exceptional capacity to "take it." Even the hardiest trainers practice negative reps only for some of their exercises and only some of the time. Negative reps require more recuperation time and can lead to some mighty sore muscles if you are not accustomed to heavy exercise, so take it easy when first trying this advanced technique.

The Pre-Exhaust System

The pre-exhaust system is based on attacking a specific muscle with a carefully chosen isolation exercise, followed immediately by a combination movement. Fitness expert, Robert Kennedy, invented this principle in the '60s.

Let's look at the chest muscles. In many chest exercises the triceps are the weak link. In dips and presses, the triceps are worked hard but the pectorals only moderately, so the triceps reach failure more rapidly than the chest. If this holds you back from developing your pectorals, the pre-exhaust method will help.

To avoid using the triceps, isolate and exhaust the pecs first by doing an exercise in which the triceps are not directly involved, such as dumbell flyes. Perform the exercise to the point of failure and go right to a combination exercise, such as the incline or bench press. After the flyes, the triceps will be temporarily stronger than the pectorals, and so will not hold your chest back in the presses.

PRE-EXHAUST

Shoulders ▶▶▶▶

ISOLATION MOVEMENT:
Lateral Raises with Dumbells (page 171)
COMBINATION MOVEMENT:
Presses Behind Neck (page 173)
or Upright Rows (page 171)

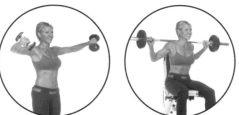

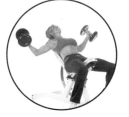 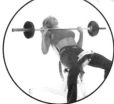

◀◀◀◀ ## Chest

ISOLATION MOVEMENT:
Incline Flyes (page 130)
COMBINATION MOVEMENT:
Bench Presses (page 128)
or Incline Bench Presses (page 128)

Quads ▶▶▶▶

ISOLATION MOVEMENT:
Leg Extensions (page 137)
COMBINATION MOVEMENT:
Squats (page 136)

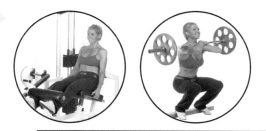

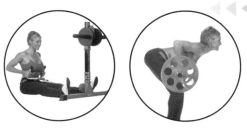

◀◀◀◀ ## Back

ISOLATION MOVEMENT:
Seated Row (page 180)
COMBINATION MOVEMENT:
Bent-Over Barbell Rows (page 177)

TIP

Prepare to be truly amazed by the power of weight training. It creates desirable curves and shapes in the most effective way.

COMBINATIONS

Abbdominals ▶▶▶▶

ISOLATION MOVEMENT:
Bench Crunches (page 165)
COMBINATION MOVEMENT:
Hanging Leg Raises (page 162)

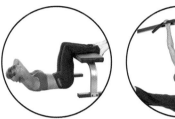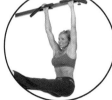

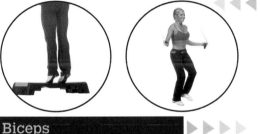

Biceps ▶▶▶▶

ISOLATION MOVEMENT:
Preacher-Bench Curls (page 155)
COMBINATION MOVEMENT:
Narrow-Undergrip Chins (page 179)

Calves ◀◀◀◀

ISOLATION MOVEMENT:
Calf Raises (page 141)
COMBINATION MOVEMENT:
Rope Jumping

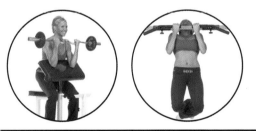

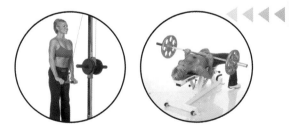

Triceps ◀◀◀◀

ISOLATION MOVEMENT:
Triceps Pressdowns (page 148)
or Single-Arm Dumbell Extensions (page 150)
COMBINATION MOVEMENT:
Close-Grip Bench Presses (page 150)

Forearms ▶▶▶▶

ISOLATION MOVEMENT:
Reverse Wrist Curls (page 157)
COMBINATION MOVEMENT:
Reverse Curls (page 157)

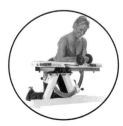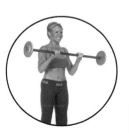

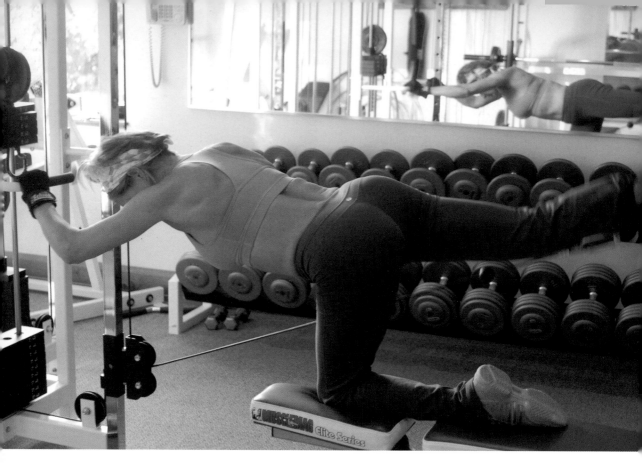

If you wish to split this routine so you train four or five times a week working only half the schedule at one time, you should work legs, back, and biceps one day, and chest, shoulders, triceps, and forearms on alternate days. The abs can be worked every day.

The number of sets and reps you do is entirely up to you. Those new to pre-exhaust training should perhaps limit their sets to two. As your condition improves you may perform up to four sets of each exercise but no more. Keep your reps around 8 to 12 per set. Many women use the pre-exhaust system on only one or two exercises in their schedule, electing to use straight sets or other variations for the balance of their training routines. A complete routine consisting entirely of pre-exhaust combinations is very demanding.

Rest-Pause Training

This method has been used since the invention of barbells. Rest-pause training is not a system to follow all the time but it does permit you to greatly increase tendon and muscle strength and add overall size in a few weeks, if that is what you want.

It's a simple idea. After warming up for a particular exercise, load up the barbell sufficiently to allow for just one repetition. Perform one difficult rep. Place the weight down, allow 10 to 20 seconds to elapse, and perform another repetition. After a similar brief rest, perform yet another repetition – and so on. After every rep you allow your body to partially recuperate. You may have to reduce the weight slightly as the reps accumulate.

Peripheral Heart Action (PHA) Training

Developed by physical educator Bob Gadja in the '60s, Peripheral Heart Action (PHA) training calls for the performance of one exercise for each major body part with a minimum of rest for four to six different areas. As you progress from one exercise to another, select movements that work totally unrelated areas. You would not, for example, perform a bench press, then a standing press, followed by dips and arm movements. Instead you might go from presses behind neck to front squats to barbell curls to calf raises. In this way the blood does not become congested in one area. Truth to tell, this may not be as effective in creating muscle stimulation as other more forceful methods, but PHA is a healthy way to train. It incorporates progressive resistance (you add weight when you can). It utilizes time well – there is no need for rest periods of any length because you are not waiting for a muscle area to partially recover before working it again, so this may be a good method for those under great time constraints.

To do a PHA routine, select four to six exercises for totally different body parts and place them into "cycles." The entire routine would then consist of two, three, or four cycles of four to six exercises each cycle. Start your cycle by performing exercise number one, then exercise number two, three, and so on. At the end of the first cycle you are permitted a two-minute rest, after which you start at the beginning of that same cycle again, or cycle two, etc.

IMPORTANT

Beginners should perform only one or two cycles. Intermediates can perform three cycles. Advanced trainers may perform up to five cycles.

BEGINNER'S ROUTINE
(Perform one or two cycles only.)

Cycle One

Bench Presses	10 reps
Barbell Curls	10 reps
Squats	12 reps
Seated Dumbell Presses	12 reps

Cycle Two

Bent-Over Barbell Rows	10 reps
Calf Raises (Standing)	10 reps
Crunches	20 reps
Straight-Arm Pullovers	12 reps
Triceps Extensions (Lying)	10 reps

INTERMEDIATE ROUTINE

(Perform three cycles.)

Cycle One

Dumbell Presses	8 reps
Squats	10 reps
Bench Presses	12 reps
Calf Raises	8 reps

Cycle Two

Leg Extensions	12 reps
Wide-Grip Pulldowns	20 reps
Hanging Leg Raises	20 reps
Barbell Curls	8 reps

Cycle Three

Incline Flyes	10 reps
Leg Curls	15 reps
Captain's Chair Sit-Ups	20 reps
Triceps Extensions (Lying)	10 reps

ADVANCED ROUTINE

(Perform three to five cycles.)

Cycle One

Standing Dumbell Presses	6 reps
Leg Curls	12 reps
Front Squats (heels on two-inch block)	10 reps
Wide-Grip Bench Presses	8 reps

Cycle Two

Captain's Chair Sit-Ups	25 reps
Bent-Over Rows	20 reps
Calf Raises	10 reps
Incline Rear Laterals	10 reps

Cycle Three

Behind-Back Wrist Curls	15 reps
Barbell Curls	10 reps
Donkey Calf Raises	25 reps
Standing Triceps Stretches	10 reps

Cycle Four

Leg Extensions	12 reps
Alternate Dumbell Curls	10 reps
Standing Lateral Raises	10 reps
Lying Triceps Extensions	10 reps

Cycle Five

Stiff-Leg Dead Lifts	12 reps
Wide-Grip Pulldowns	12 reps
Wrist Curls	15 reps
Hanging Leg Raises	20 reps

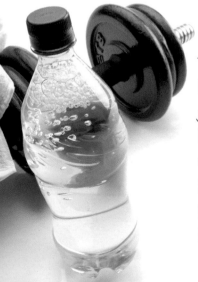

PHA Training is intense! Have your water bottle at the ready so you can keep yourself hydrated between cycles.

Giant Sets

Sometimes known as compound training, a giant set is an advanced technique for shocking your muscles into performance if they have not been responding. You perform three or four exercises for the same muscle, one after the other in rotation, with minimal rest between each exercise. *You might do:*

Barbell Curls	**10 reps**
Incline Dumbell Curls	**10 reps**
Preacher Bench Curls	**10 reps**

After you have performed one set of each of the above, go back again to the beginning and perform another cycle, or rotation. You may do two, three, or even four cycles of these giant sets, bearing in mind, of course, that four cycles would give you a total of 12 sets overall for one body part. This is definitely advanced training.

Muscle-Priority System

This is one of the oldest principles of all, one that has been highly promoted in *Oxygen* and its brother publications *MuscleMag International* and *Reps!*

You inevitably are freshest and have more vigor and energy at the beginning of a workout. Consequently, it would make sense to work whichever body part is in most need of attention first.

If you have weak, underdeveloped shoulders, for example, perform all your shoulder work first in your workout while you have the best mental drive and fresh energy to do maximum justice to the area. This may sound like common sense, but you would be surprised at how many trainers work their best areas first and their least-responsive body parts last – then they wonder why those muscles are not responding!

Peak Contraction

Very few exercises allow for full resistance to be placed on a muscle when it is completely contracted. For example, when you do a barbell curl the hardest part of the movement is when the forearms are parallel to the floor, not at the top of the curl. Peak contraction is the term used to describe movements for which the hardest part of an exercise coincides with the muscle being fully contracted. As Robert Kennedy says in his book *MuscleBuilding*: *"To get the most out of an exercise, you should have a heavy weight on a working muscle when the largest number of muscle cells are being fired off."*

The peak-contraction training principle keeps stress on the muscle when it is fully contracted. Some of these exercises are: 90-degree preacher bench curls, incline or standing leg curls, leg extensions, hyperextensions, shrugs, calf raises, upright rows, bent-over rows, pulldowns, side laterals, dumbell kickbacks, crunches, bent-over laterals, front barbell and dumbell laterals, supine dumbell curls, hanging leg raises, and inversion boot sit-ups.

When you employ peak-contraction exercises you should consciously hold the fully contracted position of each repetition for two or three seconds to maximally engage all the muscle fibers.

Pyramid Training

Pyramid training is used by pro bodybuilders more than any other principle. It involves adding weight and decreasing repetitions with each successive set. After your heaviest weight has been used, there is a corresponding reduction (or stripping) in weight for each successive set as you gradually work back down. The pyramid method is almost always used in the squat and bench press.

Here's how a particular pyramid set might work out for you in the squat.

SET 1	40 lbs, 20 reps
SET 2	80 lbs, 12 reps
SET 3	100 lbs, 10 reps
SET 4	120 lbs, 8 reps
SET 5	130 lbs, 6 reps
SET 6	100 lbs, 15 reps
SET 7	80 lbs, 20 reps

The first two sets are little more than warm-ups for the "work" sets that follow.

We have now covered all the major resistance-training principles and exercises you should know – whether you are just getting started or are determined to become a top contender in fitness competition. Just how far you wish to go is entirely up to you. If you are a beginner to progressive-resistance exercise, a simple routine involving straight sets is just fine.

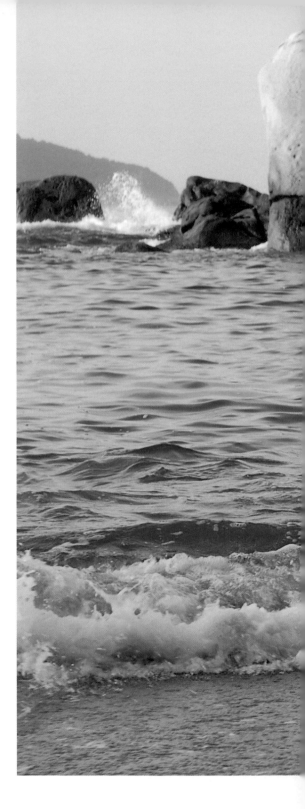

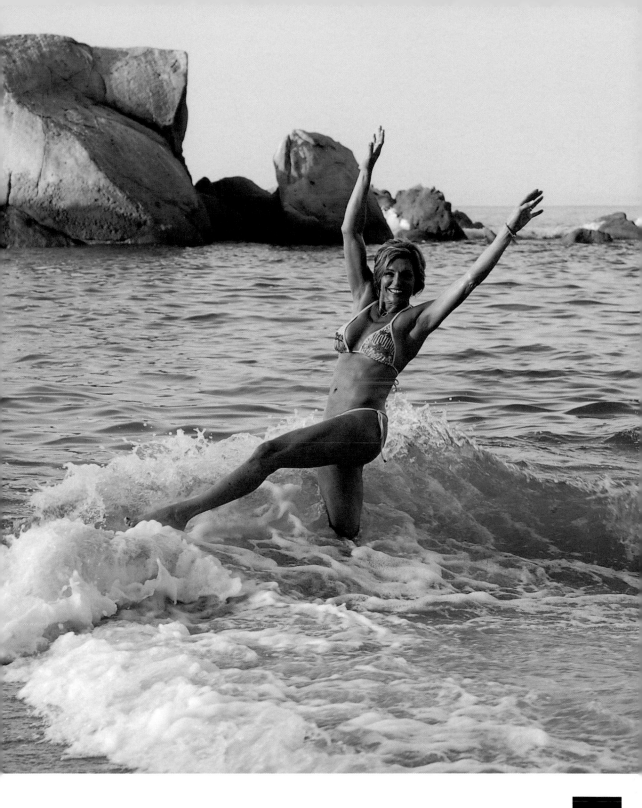

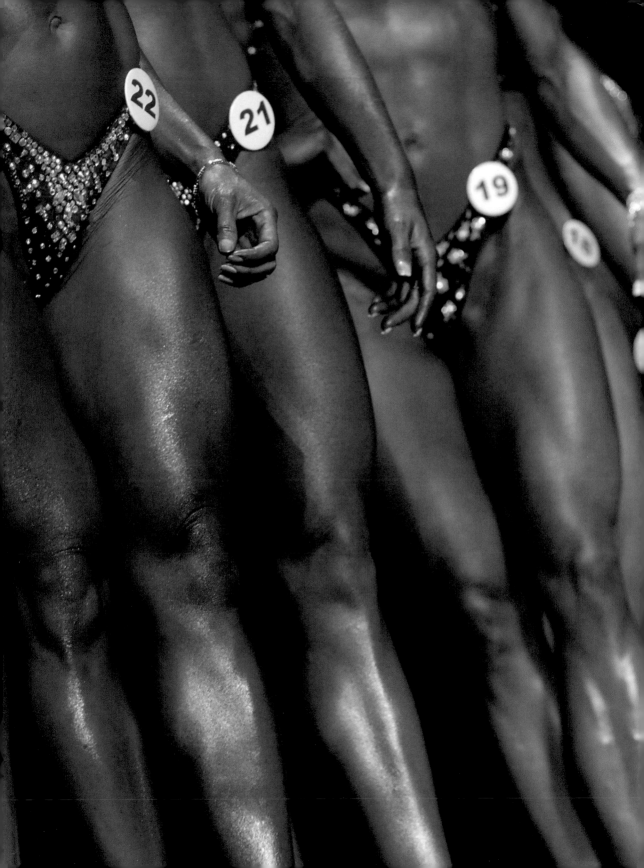

17

Did you know you can get judged on your new physique? Competition is a great way to get rewarded for all of your hard work! Read on for the next step in training.

GETTING RIPPED
PEAK PREPARATION

Getting "ripped" is a process in which a fitness trainer reduces her body-fat level to show her muscles to maximum effect for a special event, a wedding, a photo session, a contest, etc. This is primarily done with diet and aerobic exercise. Your actual weight-training schedule should include more isolation exercises (movements that involve only one joint) than you would normally use during regular training. As peak time approaches, your exercises can be performed with increased intensity and with somewhat less rest between sets.

How low should your body-fat percentage go? Most women aim to weigh in at 10 to 12 percent body fat. You may hear of lower percentages, but these are seldom documented. Besides, too low is too low.

Many people make the mistake of dieting too late and too drastically. An extreme reduction in calories will set off a physiological alarm, directing the body to rebel and retain fat cells. Your metabolic rate will quickly lower to compensate for the "coming famine." Your body will begin storing calories as fat and you will become smoother – the exact opposite of what you want.

One fitness competitor says: "I never starve myself before competition. Four months before a big show such as the IFBB Ms. Olympia Fitness, I reduce my calories slightly. At this stage I am only eight or nine pounds over my best contest weight. I just do not believe in bulking (fattening) up in the off-season. I take those eight pounds off at the rate of just eight ounces a week (two pounds a month) and I believe this is the only sensible way to reduce." I tend to follow that advice as well. I hate to get too far away from my ideal weight. I'd rather keep as tight as I can most of the time and step things up but not too drastically for the big event, whatever it may be.

During the last four months before the time I want to peak my diet begins to get stringent. I still eat six meals a day, each consisting of lean protein and complex carbohydrates, but I begin to rely heavily on leafy green and fibrous veggies such as green beans and asparagus. I understand the value of creating lean muscle with the help of healthy fats: flaxseed, pumpkinseed, and raw unsalted nuts.

The average woman carries about 25 to 30 percent body fat, while the average man has 15 to 20 percent. A woman who lowers her body fat to 10 to 12 percent will look extremely lean and muscular. Some women have been known to go lower – even down to four percent! However, we must ask ourselves if less is always better.

Low body fat is important for winning a contest, but if you go too low you will appear stringy and emaciated, which detracts from your appearance. Besides, only a small percentage of women want to enter contests. Most of us just want to look attractive in a bikini. It's nice to have toned-looking muscles at the beach but bulging, ripped-to-shreds, vein-choked freaky development is not something I strive for, that's for sure.

A woman's menstrual cycle is disrupted when her body fat goes too low. This absence of periods (amenorrhea) is nature's precaution against a woman getting pregnant when she doesn't appear to have the nutritional supply to support the healthy growth of a fetus.

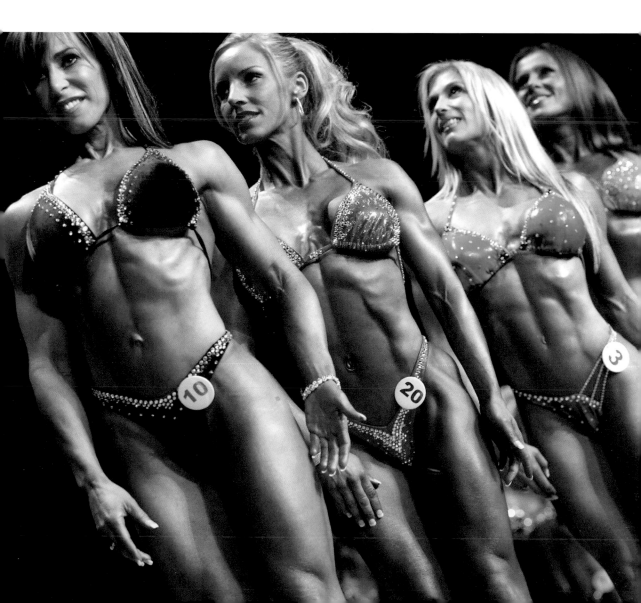

TIP

"Getting ripped is a process requiring serious motivation. If you can't say no to Twinkies this is not for you!"

"There is no evidence to show that temporary amenorrhea is harmful to the female reproductive system," concluded the American College of Sports Medicine in a recent study after recognizing the fact that many female athletes had menstrual irregularities as a result of achieving low body fat levels. If you experience amenorrhea when competing, then make sure to bring your body-fat level up to regain your natural menstural cycle. Long-term amenorrhea can be detrimental to skeletal density.

When you reduce your body-fat level your breasts will also lose considerable size (being primarily made up of fat cells). During peak conditioning women have a minimum of breast adipose tissue. Sorry about that news, but it is absolutely inevitable.

Salt is one of the dietary enemies of ripping up. Table salt is the biggest offender, but if you study labels you will be surprised at how much there is in most prepared foods. Fitness aspirants will often be quite liberal with their salt intake until the last four or five days. Then they absolutely stop all salt intake in order to avoid water retention at contest time. If a woman tries to keep salt out of her diet for more than a few days, weeks, or even months, then even the smallest slip can result in a high degree of water retention. Fitness pro Monica Brant agrees with this philosophy. You cannot avoid salt for too long a period.

Diuretics are used by some women in order to induce the body to shed water via excessive urination. This is definitely a dangerous practice

since it can deplete potassium stores in the body. Along with other jobs, potassium is responsible for keeping your heartbeat regular. Without it you could suffer cardiac arrest. Avoid using harsh drugstore or prescription diuretics, at all costs.

One expert believes that it is a good idea to reward yourself with a healthy serving of high-fat foods every five or six days while on a strict diet. "A couple of scoops of ice cream makes a perfect diversion," they say. "It will help you keep your sanity without wrecking your weight-loss momentum." My advice is: Let's make it every 10 to 12 days.

TIP

I stick to healthy fats from nutritious sources. My faves include unsalted raw nuts, flaxseed and natural nut butters.

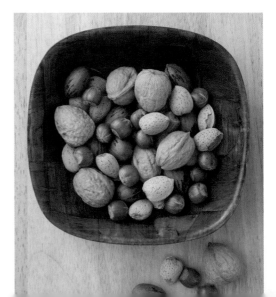

If you are entering a contest the final days are hardest because you must make that extra effort to restrict food intake while still trying to maximize workout intensity so that muscle is not lost. At such times you will find yourself running out of steam in the middle of workouts and wondering if it is all worth it. Resist the temptation to throw in the towel at this point. Remember, the stage is not full of hundreds of women doing what you are doing – you are among a select few who can push themselves this hard.

During the last 10 days, reduce your carbohydrate intake to 80 grams daily, dropping down to about 50 grams daily for the last six days. Then during the last 24 to 36 hours before being judged you should increase your carbohydrate consumption. This is known as carbohydrate loading (carbing up!). When this method is correctly used, you will get full-looking muscles and sharp definition. Some successful competitors prefer to carb up slowly during the last three days prior to competition, rather than risk too much from a one-day binge just before the show. This is a matter for your own experimentation.

Make sure you carb up with complex carbohydrates such as a sweet potato or brown rice rather than resorting to sugar, ice cream or even fruit. Also, if you eat too much you run into the danger of accumulating excess water beneath the skin. During the last two days you should drink only enough liquids to quench your thirst on a short-term basis. Competitors normally drink distilled water, which has minimal sodium, if any.

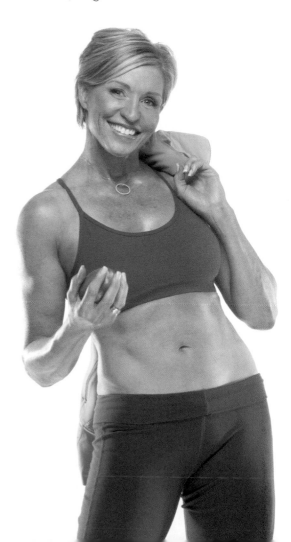

TIP

Remember that contest dieting is not an exact science. What works for me does not necessarily work for others. You need to play with your nutrition to get it right for you.

CONTEST DOS AND DON'TS

For those who have it in the back of their mind that they would like to one day try their luck at competing, here are a few rules:

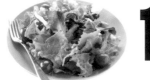

1

Do make sure that you start your diet well in advance of the contest – at least three or four months is optimal.

Do not cut calorie consumption drastically in the hope of getting into top shape in a week or two. This will only set you up for disaster.

2

3

Do get a good natural tan in the months leading up to a contest. Make sure you tan evenly, including under your arms. Most women also use an artificial tanning product, which is applied daily during the last week or two before a contest. Build up layers of artificial tan to get an overall dark and even tan.

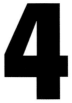

Do be totally prepared for a show. Take along a sweatsuit, sneakers, two costumes, tanning lotion for last-minute touch-ups, towel, oil, shower slippers, music, stage pass and your makeup and grooming kit. And please don't forget to pack your dazzling smile!

4

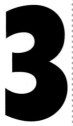

5

Do not enter a contest unless you are ready for it. Attend several contests before you enter one as a competitor to learn what is expected of you. If you compete at a level way above your head you will only feel foolish and possibly embarrassed.

Do not compete in too many contests. You can peak only two or three times a year at the most. An overabundance of contests could burn you out.

6

7

Do not cover your body with excessive amounts of oil. Apply vegetable oil (almond or avocado) and not a petroleum-based oil, which will appear too reflective. Vegetable oil sinks into the skin. Make sure to apply the oil evenly, so there are no "hot spots" or areas that are so slick with oil they become reflective. Do not compete without any oil.

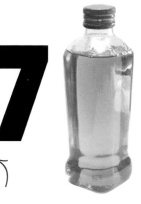

TIP

Pam is the spray-on oil most competitors prefer. It may stink, but it works. I like the olive oil-based version.

8

Do not pump up excessively (floor dips, chins, light dumbell work) before going on stage. This will flatten out your physique. Merely perform a few exercises to get the blood circulating so you can feel your muscles. Work only those areas that need a little more size. Do not pump up your legs. Doing so would interfere with your sensitivity for posing and no visible difference will be noticed from your efforts.

9

Do be alive, alert, and ready. You are being looked at, assessed and appraised onstage. Even when the judges are assessing other women you should keep your muscles semi-tensed – you never know when a judge might look back at you. Even if you aren't completely comfortable, pretend that you are. Be aware of directives from the head judge. Know your number as well as the order of any compulsory poses required.

10

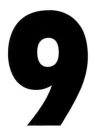

Do smile when you're onstage. This is show business, and it takes showmanship to win. You have to think of yourself as a performer. I have seen many a perfect physique ruined by a poor attitude and lack of sparkle in the face. You must sell yourself the best you possibly can. Oh, yes – and good luck!

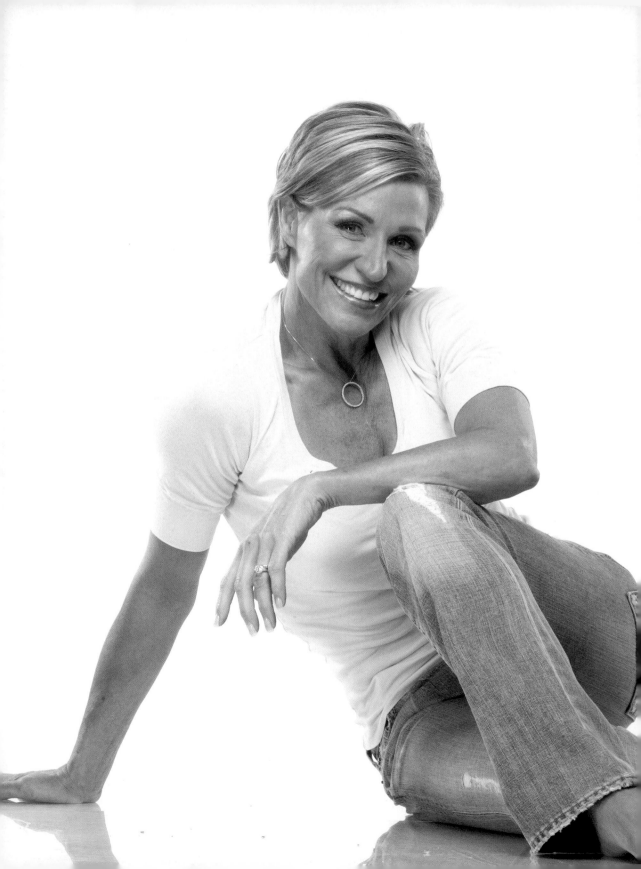

18

"There are no shortcuts to any place worth going."

BEVERLY SILLS

QUESTIONS & ANSWERS

Q.

CAN I STILL TRAIN EVEN IF I AM PREGNANT?

A.

Many women find if they are already reasonably fit and in the habit of training, they can keep up with training throughout most of the pregnancy. Whether or not you can depends very much on your fitness level, how hard you are currently training, and also on your level of health during your pregnancy.

Paula Radcliffe, the marathoner from Britain, managed to keep up with her almost superhuman levels of endurance training throughout her pregnancy, delivered a healthy baby and then went right back to training. She was physically and mentally prepared for this.

You definitely don't have to give up on training and fitness altogether just because you are pregnant, unless you have a health issue that causes your doctor to prescribe bed rest. However, this is not the ideal time to begin a tough training program or decide to lose weight. This flies in the face of logic and logic is precisely what you should rely on during this exciting time of life.

It is a well-known fact that if you have trained throughout your pregnancy chances are very good you will not gain excess weight and that whatever you did gain will come off quickly. Do avoid getting overheated when exercising, though, as overheating can cause damage to your baby.

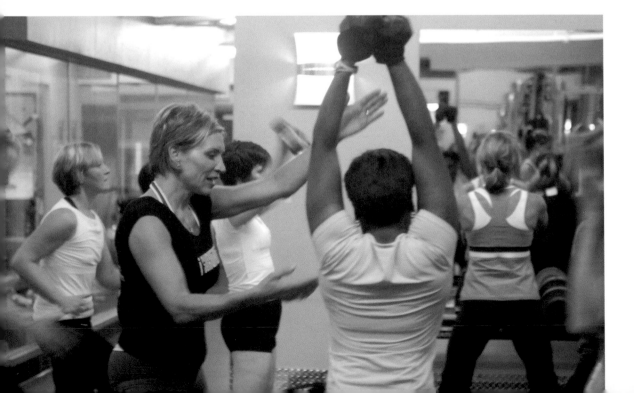

Q.

CAN I STILL TRAIN IF I AM SICK OR INJURED?

A.

Some of us get so involved with training we want to keep up with it even when we are either injured or sick. This is another one of those situations where you will need to use your head and let the voice of reason coach you onwards. Obviously if you are deathly ill there is no benefit to training. You simply will not have the energy or the stamina to do it properly. Even worse, you could cause your situation to deteriorate, or you could make others around you sick. So don't even consider it.

You can train if you are just recovering from some sort of elective surgery that doesn't require you to be bedridden. I can think of one time when I had a minor corrective procedure on my foot. Even with the air cast on I could do some weight training and a bit of walking. You can also train around an injured body part. Your own situation regarding health and degree of injury or illness should guide you. And look at it this way: sometimes a forced rest is a fabulous way to take a break and recharge your fitness batteries.

Q.

I TREAT MYSELF SOMETIMES AND HAVE MORE CAKE AND ICE CREAM THAN I SHOULD. THE WAY I FIX THIS IS TO DO A FEW EXTRA HOURS OF CARDIO. AM I KIDDING MYSELF?

A.

You get a resounding YES! in answer to this. If there is one pervasive myth out there about burning off unwanted calories, this is it. At one time or another we have all followed this misguided idea and it just does not work. Ever! You can't chase unwanted calories by charging up your treadmill and hoping the session will erase your indulgence. Whatever food you take in, it is processed in a normal fashion. All macronutrients are treated equally once they arrive in your stomach. There is no back door for the hunk of carrot cake you ate. It must be processed the same way protein gets processed. However, the higher the quality of your nutrition, the more efficiently these foods will burn. The more processed and refined your food is, the more complicated the process and the more junk you will store as fat.

Q.

I HEAR ABOUT PEOPLE TAKING A WEEK-LONG BREAK FROM TRAINING TO GIVE THEIR MUSCLES A REST. IS THIS NECESSARY?

A.

It is true that even the most seasoned weight-trained athlete will take a break from training. Depending on how hard you are driving yourself a break like this can do wonders. Some people feel it recharges their battery while others feel it helps them remember why they love the training lifestyle so much. It is not absolutely necessary to take a break like this but if you feel you are struggling and need to, then please do so. This may be particularly applicable when you are traveling and far from a dumbell or gym.

Q.

ONE SIDE OF MY BODY IS NOT THE SAME AS THE OTHER. I NOTICE THAT I AM NOT COMPLETELY SYMMETRICAL. HOW CAN I FIX THIS?

A.

Relax! The fact that you are asymmetrical means you are human and very normal. Virtually everyone has some degree of asymmetry and most of the time it is hardly noticeable. It is true when you are competing that symmetry is one of the judging criteria and the pros have to try and overcome nature. What this means is they spend a little time correcting the under-built area. If the left biceps is smaller than the right, do a few more reps on the left to try to push the muscle into growth. Another way of improving asymmetry is to visit a chiropractor. You may have a particular skeletal imbalance. Most of the time, though, there is nothing to worry about!

Q.

I HAVE NOTICED THAT PROPORTION IS A CONCERN WHEN TRAINING. SOME PEOPLE HAVE HUGE LEGS AND THEN NO ARMS. HOW DO YOU ADDRESS PROPORTION?

A.

Proportion is of more concern than symmetry. Since everyone has some degree of asymmetry and it is often hardly noticeable, you can virtually ignore it unless you are planning to compete. However, it is pretty obvious if someone has completely trained legs but no abs or arms to speak of. The way to avoid this trap is to start your training session with the weakest muscle group. This is called muscle priority. Giving those trouble spots priority when you are

Me with my training buddy Franca Jarullo.
Love it! Love it! Love it!

freshest means you will give them 100 percent right at the start. Leaving them to the end may put you in a position where you are tempted to either train them less rigorously or not at all. Women tend to be more proportion minded than men. We accept that our bodies have weak spots and don't mind working harder to achieve balance.

Q.

I AM SERIOUS ABOUT WEIGHT TRAINING BUT FREQUENTLY HAVE TO SPEND ONE WEEK IN A HOTEL WHERE THERE ARE NO GYM FACILITIES. WHAT CAN I DO?

A.

When I traveled to the South Pacific recently I could not find a gym anywhere. Luckily there are hundreds of exercises you can do using your own body weight as resistance. Chins are a great example. They work your lats and other back muscles. Then there are squats, lunges, pushups, crunches and standing calf raises. I even rigged up a towel from a beam in the hotel room and did triceps and biceps exercises. One can be very creative when necessary! I like the challenge of devising ways to train muscles without the standard equipment. In any case, you can make it work if you are hungry to keep up with your training.

Q.

IT'S HARD TO KNOW WHAT I AM SUPPOSED TO EAT BEFORE AND AFTER A WORKOUT. WHAT DO YOU RECOMMEND?

A.

It is easy to get hung up about what to eat and when and how it relates to training. Let's try to remember that the first rule of Clean Eating is eating every three hours. That means eating has to fit into your training schedule. Now I don't suggest bringing your lunch entrée into the gym, but there are ways to eat that make sense. The rule of thumb for eating around a workout is to eat for energy before a workout and eat for muscle repair after a workout. Energy foods would be those loaded with complex carbohydrates that translate into ready fuel soon after ingestion. You might consider a banana and a handful of unsalted, raw almonds and a glass of water as a pre-workout option. Foods containing protein are excellent for muscle repair. Many people like to have a protein shake after a workout. Whatever you choose, if you have just had a small Clean-Eating meal, wait for 30 minutes before you train.

SO MANY MODELS IN *OXYGEN* MAGAZINE LOOK LIKE THEY SPEND HOURS AND HOURS IN THE GYM, INCLUDING YOU. HOW LONG DO YOU REALLY TRAIN?

A.

I love to train, but I am no fool. I enjoy it because I know I can get excellent results in little time. On any given training day I work two or three body parts. I like to mix it up every workout, but I generally pick two exercises for each of those body parts unless I am training legs, in which case I do three exercises. I perform 5 sets of 10 to 15 repetitions (reps) for each of these exercises. I like to train until I feel the Sweet Pain. That's a good clue – go to where it feels like you are definitely training, but not over the edge. Most of my training sessions last about 45 minutes. Then I do some stretching and I am out the door. I'll do cardio four times per week but I don't spend hours on the treadmill – only 35 minutes or so. It's not about how much, it's about how good. Quality is your friend! Remember training is a privilege, not a punishment.

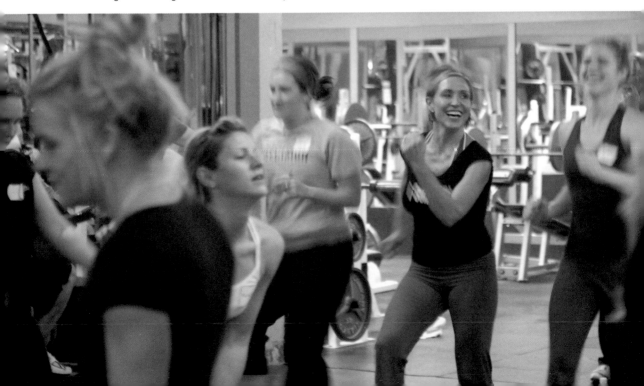

YOUR TRAINING
JOURNAL

DATE

BODY PART	EXERCISE		SET 1	SET 2	SET 3	SET 4	SET 5
		WEIGHT					
		REPS					
		WEIGHT					
		REPS					
		WEIGHT					
		REPS					
		WEIGHT					
		REPS					
		WEIGHT					
		REPS					
		WEIGHT					
		REPS					
		WEIGHT					
		REPS					
		WEIGHT					
		REPS					

CARDIO ACTIVITY:

NOTES:

YOUR TRAINING
JOURNAL

DATE

BODY PART	EXERCISE		SET 1	SET 2	SET 3	SET 4	SET 5
		WEIGHT					
		REPS					
		WEIGHT					
		REPS					
		WEIGHT					
		REPS					
		WEIGHT					
		REPS					
		WEIGHT					
		REPS					
		WEIGHT					
		REPS					
		WEIGHT					
		REPS					
		WEIGHT					
		REPS					

CARDIO ACTIVITY:

NOTES:

GOALS

Setting goals is the key to success. Each goal is a stepping stone toward your ideal self. Give yourself reasonable goals to work toward. Rather than trying to lose 20 lbs. in one week, strive for 2 lbs. You can try for 20 lbs. over time.

Breaking your long-term goal into attainable short-term goals keeps you aware of your progress, and you are constantly rewarding yourself by completing one step toward a better you!

WEEKLY GOALS

Making positive changes each week will add up. You'll start seeing results in no time!
By this time next week...

MONTHLY GOALS

Some of your goals will take a little longer. Choose a few monthly goals and stick to the changes you've already made.
By this time next month...

LONG-TERM GOALS

Studies have shown that people who write down their long-term goals are more successful in many aspects of life than those who do not. Do it now!
By this time next year...

GOALS

Setting goals is the key to success. Each goal is a stepping stone toward your ideal self. Give yourself reasonable goals to work toward. Rather than trying to lose 20 lbs. in one week, strive for 2 lbs. You can try for 20 lbs. over time.

Breaking your long-term goal into attainable short-term goals keeps you aware of your progress, and you are constantly rewarding yourself by completing one step toward a better you!

WEEKLY GOALS

Making positive changes each week will add up. You'll start seeing results in no time!
By this time next week...

MONTHLY GOALS

Some of your goals will take a little longer. Choose a few monthly goals and stick to the changes you've already made.
By this time next month...

LONG-TERM GOALS

Studies have shown that people who write down their long-term goals are more successful in many aspects of life than those who do not. Do it now!
By this time next year...

A

Abdominals (abs): this muscle group is composed of the rectus abdominis, transversus abdominis, and the external and internal obliques. It forms the abdomen of the body and acts as a torso flexor and rotator.

Aerobic exercise: exercise for which the body uses oxygen in order to burn required energy. Also: steady-state rhythmic exercises that tax the aerobic system, thereby improving the oxygen consumption of the body.

Amenorrhea: the absence of menstrual periods often caused by low-body fat percentage and low caloric intake.

Amino acids: called the "building blocks of life," amino acids are biochemical subunits linked together by chemical bonds to form polypeptide chains. Hundreds of polypeptides, in turn, link together to form a protein molecule.

Anaerobic exercise: any high-intensity exercise that outstrips the body's aerobic capacity and leads to an oxygen debt. Because of its intensity, anaerobic exercise can be maintained for only short periods of time.

Asymmetric training: any exercise that targets only one side of the body. Single-arm dumbell curls, lateral raises and single-arm triceps extensions are all examples of asymmetric training.

B

Ballistic stretching: stretching with bouncing movements.

Barbell: a steel bar typically five to seven feet in length that may be used on its own or with sleeve, collar and plate attachments for resistance training. They may be either fixed (the plates are kept in place by welded collars) or adjustable (allowing the changing of plates).

Biceps: a two-headed muscle that makes up the front of the arm and acts as an elbow flexor.

Bodybuilder: an individual who uses nutrition and exercise to create an aesthetically pleasing physique – sometimes in order to compete in bodybuilding contests.

Body fat: a body tissue specialized to contain high-energy oils which act as an energy reserve.

Body-fat percentage: the ratio of fat to bodyweight. For most women, seventeen to twenty percent is ideal.

Buttocks: another term referring to the gluteus maximus, medius and minimus.

C

Cadence: the rhythm and sequence of a series of actions, such as repetitions of an exercise.

Carbohydrate loading: the practice of depleting and replenishing the body's glycogen levels in the weeks leading up to a bodybuilding contest. This technique allows bodybuilders to saturate their muscles with stored water, thus making the muscles fuller and harder.

Cardiovascular training: exercise that taxes the heart and lungs to improve their function.

Cheating: executing a movement without proper form, to make it easier.

Chelated mineral supplement: a type of supplement whereby the mineral is firmly attached to an organic compound, such as an amino acid, so the molecules do not dissociate in the digestive system and are better absorbed by the body.

Chest: the large pectoral muscles located on the front of the upper torso, responsible for drawing the arms towards the center of the body.

Circuit training: a specialized form of weight training that combines strength training and aerobic conditioning. Circuit training consists of performing 10 to 20 different exercises, one after the other, with little rest between sets.

Clean Eating: a diet consisting of all-natural lean proteins, complex carbohydrates from whole grains, fruits and vegetables, and healthy fats eaten in combination every two to three hours.

Clear vision: knowing your needs and desires and how to translate them into reality without wasting energy on anxiety.

Compound exercises: any exercise working more than one muscle group. Popular compound movements include bench presses, squats, shoulder presses and bent-over rows.

Concentric: a type of contraction whereby the muscle shortens to generate force.

Contraction: the generation of tension by muscle fibers.

Cut: competitive term used to describe the physical appearance of a physique competitor. To be "cut" implies that you are in great competitive shape, with extremely low body-fat levels.

D

Deltoid: Muscle that encapsulates the shoulder. This muscle has three heads: the anterior, lateral and posterior.

Density: term used to describe the mass of a substance for a particular area. Example: a body is denser if it has more muscle mass than fat mass.

Dietary fat: fat present in food. It is responsible for the carriage of fat-soluble vitamins into the system, the maintenance of healthy skin and hair, protection of organs, insulation and satiety after meals.

Dietary Reference Intake (DRI): the estimated average requirement (EAR), reference daily intake (RDI), adequate intake (AI), and tolerable upper intake levels (UL) for each nutrient are summed up in the DRI. This system is used in both the US and Canada.

Duiretic: any natural or synthetic chemical that causes the body to excrete water. In most cases the drug interacts with aldosterone, the hormone responsible for water retention. Diuretics also flush electrolytes from the body, which is very dangerous.

Dumbell: a handheld object that comes in a variety of weights and shapes, used for resistance training. Also spelled dumbbell.

Dynamic stretching: rhythmic stretching.

E

Eccentric: contraction whereby the muscle lengthens while garnering force.

Endurance: the ability to maintain an activity for a length of time.

Erector spinae (erectors): stabilizing muscles that run along either side of the spinal column. They are powerful spinal flexors.

Exercise: in general terms, any form of physical activity that increases the heart and respiratory rate. In bodybuilding terms, an exercise is one specific movement for one or more muscle groups.

F

Fast-twitch muscle fiber: a muscle fiber that is adapted for rapid, short-duration contractions.

Fat: see body fat or dietary fat

Flexibility: The range of motion of joints.

Free weights: term given to barbells and dumbells. Free-weight exercises are the most popular types performed by bodybuilders.

Frequency: the number of times you perform your workout routine.

G

Gastrocnemius (calf): found at the back of the lower leg, this muscle is involved in ankle plantar flexion (pushing your toes down) and slight knee flexion.

Glutes: comprised of the gluteus minimus, gluteus medius, and large gluteus maximus, this muscle group composes the backside of the body (your rear-end, or buttocks) and serves as a powerful hip extensor, external rotator, abductor and knee flexor.

H

Hamstrings: three muscles (biceps femoris, semimembranosus and semitendinosus) that serve to flex the knee joint and make up the back of the upper leg.

High Intensity Interval Training (HIITs): cardiovascular training that involves both anaerobic and aerobic training by using periods of both high and low intensity.

I

Injuries: physical injuries include any damage to bone, muscle or connective tissue. The most common bodybuilding injuries are muscle strains.

Intensity: the degree of difficulty involved in an exercise.

Intercostals: small, finger-like muscles located along the sides of the lower abdomen, between the rib cage and the obliques.

Iron pills: a slang term used to describe weights.

Isolation exercises: any exercise aimed at working only one muscle. In most cases, it's virtually impossible to totally isolate a muscle. Some common examples are: preacher curls, lateral raises, and triceps pushdowns.

J

Joint: the point at which two bones meet. Most joints have a hinge-type structure that allows the bones to articulate with one another.

K

Kyphlordosis: a combination of kyphosis and lordosis.

Kyphosis (humpback): an overly rounded upper back.

L

Latissimus dorsi (lats): the fan-shaped muscles located on the back of the torso that, when properly developed, give the V-taper. The lats function to pull the arms down and back.

Ligament: connecting tissue that improves joint stability by connecting the articulating bones of a joint. For example, the anterior cruciate ligament (ACL) of the knee connects the tibia (shin bone) to the femur (thigh bone).

Lordosis (swayback): the abnormal forward tilting of the pelvis.

M

Mitochondria: as the "powerhouse" of the human cell, this organelle generates ATP, which our cells use for energy. When a muscle is trained, the density of mitochondria in that muscle will increase, making our muscle more efficient.

Muscle: contractile tissue of the body that produces the force necessary for motion of the limbs or function of internal organs.

Muscularity: the degree to which the muscles in the body are developed.

N

Negatives: also known as eccentric contractions because the muscle lengthens while still under tension. The muscle is acting as a brake to slow down the lowering of the barbell. For example, the controlled lowering of the weight back to the chest during a bench press.

Nutrition: the art of combining foods in the right amounts so the human body receives all of the required nutrients.

O

Obesity: a state of being extremely overweight (over 25% body fat for men and 30% body fat for women).

Obliques: muscles with both internal and external groups that hug the waist and allow for rotation of the torso.

Overtraining: the physiological state whereby the individual's recovery system is taxed to the limit. In many cases, insufficient time is allowed for recovery between workouts. Among the more common symptoms are: muscle loss, lack of motivation, insomnia, and reduced energy.

Oxygen debt: increased amounts of oxygen consumed following a strenuous activity in order to replenish the muscle tissue with nutrients and remove waste products.

P

Peak: this can mean the degree of sharpness or shape held by a particular muscle (usually the biceps), or it may refer to the shape a bodybuilder or fitness competitor holds on a given contest day. A woman who has "peaked" is in top condition.

Pectorals: this grouping of muscles includes the pectoralis minor and pectoralis major, to make up the chest.

Physical fitness: a general state of well-being and the ability to perform a function.

Physical stress test: the performance of a series of activities used to determine physical fitness, done under the control of a medical physician.

Plateau: a state of training in which no progress is being made. Plateaus usually occur after long periods of repetitious training. Breaking the condition involves shocking the muscles with new training techniques.

Plyometrics: exercise involving a quick eccentric phase followed by an explosive concentric phase used to generate force to develop muscular power, example: jumping.

Positives: part of the rep that goes against gravity. In barbell biceps curls, the positive phase would occur during the curling of the barbell.

Posture: position of the body.

Progressive resistance exercise: development of physical fitness using a slow, methodical program involving increased intensity as the body reaches new plateaus.

Proportion: term used to describe the size of one muscle with respect to the whole body. A bodybuilder or fitness competitor with good "proportion" would have all her muscles in balance with regards to size.

Protein: nutrient composed of long chains of amino acids. Protein is primarily used in the production of muscle tissue, hormones, and enzymes.

Q

Quadriceps: four muscles (rectus femoris, vastus medialis, vastus lateralis and vastus intermedius) that serve as powerful knee extensors, accessory hip flexors, and compose the front of the upper leg.

R

Range of motion: the distance between the flexed and extended positions of a joint.

Resistance training: forcing your muscles to work against the body, gravity, weights or other resistance in order to build strength.

Rhomboids: muscles found in the middle of the back that squeeze the shoulder blades together.

Ripped: another term to describe the percentage of body fat carried by a physique competitor. A ripped fitness competitor has a very low body-fat percentage (8 – 12%).

S

Shoulder: made up of the deltoid muscle, this area of the body is responsible for elevating the arm and rotating the shoulder girdle.

Slow-twitch muscle fiber: type of muscle fiber adapted for slow contractions of long duration.

Split training: dividing your full-body workout into separate training days.

Static stretching: holding a stretched position for a certain length of time.

Steroids: synthetic derivatives of the hormone testosterone that allow the user to gain muscle mass and strength more rapidly.

Stretching: a series of movements that stretch the joints beyond a comfortable range of motion in order to increase flexibility.

Strict form: training technique that involves performing exercises in a slow, controlled manner, and through a full range of motion, without the aid of a partner or cheating techniques.

Supplements: nutrient products (vitamin, mineral, protein or other) consumed in tablet, capsule, powder, oil or plant form to make up for a possible deficiency in the diet.

T

Tendon: tissue connecting a muscle to a bone in order to transfer the energy of the muscle to move the bone. For example, when you perform a biceps curl, the biceps tendon pulls your forearm upwards.

Testosterone: an anabolic steroid hormone, found in both male and female reproductive organs, which increases protein synthesis in order to build up muscle tissue. Male adults produce eight times more testosterone than female adults.

Trapezius (traps): the muscle that shrugs the shoulder and squeezes the shoulder blades together. It runs from the nape of the neck to the shoulder and down to the middle of the back.

Triceps: a muscle with three heads that serves to extend the elbow. It composes the back of the upper arm.

W

Warm up: any form of light, short-duration exercise that prepares the body for more intense exercise. Warming up should involve increasing the heart and respiratory rate.

A

Abdomen, 38
Abdominals (abs), 99,10-121,158-167,190
Adaptation, 50
Adock, Sonia, 59
Adrenaline, 54
Advanced, 45-46,104,112-113,114-121,188,194
Age, 22-24
Aerobic, 29-31,89,92
Aerobic workouts, 31
Air displacement plethysmography, 20
Alicia Marie, 93
Almonds, 79,83
Ambition, 58
Amenorrhea, 201-202
Amino acids, 82-83
    essential, 82
Anabolic steroids, 84-85
    side effects of, 84
Anaerobic, 89,92
Ascorbic acid, 80
Asparagus, 80
Assisted chin/dip machine, 178
Atlas, Charles, 186

B

Back, 99,116,174-183,190
Back Specialization Routine, The, 116-117
Baily, Covert, 89
Ballistic stretching, 40
Barbell (s), 65,67,70,75,128,136-137,141,146,150,156-157,81-182,92
Barbell presses,
    standing, 173
Basic Routine, The, 110
Bat wings, 21
Beans, 79
Beef, 83
Beer belly, 21
Beginners, 26,29,32-33,45,47,104,106,128,193
Beginner's Routine, The, 106
Bench, 64, 67, 70, 173
    adjustable incline, 70,128,130
    flat, 135,150,153,163,166,173
    Gironda, 74
    incline, 178
    multi-purpose, 74
    preacher, 74,156
Scott, 74
Bench presses, 106-107,109,110,114,118,121,126,128,193-194

close-grip, 71,109,150,190
flat dumbell, 130
incline, 117-118,128,152,190
medium-grip, 190
wide-grip, 99, 194
Bent-over dumbell extensions, 97
Bent-over rows, 96,99
Bent-over twists, 165
Berger, Stuart, 88
Berries,
    acai, 80
    goji, 80
Biceps, 97,106-121,144-157,190
Bioelectrical impedance (BIA), 19
Blood clotting, 80
Blood vessels, 80
Bod pod, 20
Bodybuilder, 14,20,24,71,72,154,196
Bodybuilding, 14, 44, 58
Bodybuilding supplements, 83
Body composition, 19
Body-fat percentage, 19, 25
Body mass index (BMI), 20
Bones, 79-80, 82
Bone marrow, 80
Bouncing, 37, 40
Brachialis, 146
Brant, Monica, 93,127,161
Breast(s), 126
Breast implants, 126
Breathing, 29-30, 51
Broccoli, 79-80
Brussels sprouts, 80
Buddha belly, 21
Butter, 89
Buttocks, 137

C

Cabbage, 79-80
Cable crossovers, 190
Cadence, 30
Cakes, 89
Calcium, 82
    absorption of, 80
Calf, 72
Calf machine, 142
Calf raises, 110, 190, 194
    donkey, 114,116,120,143,194
    seated, 113,119,120,142
    single-leg, 143

E

Eat Clean, 26, 92-93, 160
Eccentric contraction, 189
Egg(s), 79, 83, 93
    white(s), 83
    yolk(s), 79-80
Elbow brace, 70
Endurance, 24
Enthusiasm, 56
Erectors, 118
Estrogen, 84
Exercise, (Herbert M. Shelton, MD) 100
Exercise, 23,63
EZ-curl bar (s), 71,150

F

Fasting, 88-89
Fat, 10,18-19,21,23,26,88-89,93
    distribution of, 18
    intra-abdominal, 20
    subcutaneous, 20
Fat-free mass, 19-20
Fat loss, 26
Fat mass, 19-20
Feedback, 56
Figure skating, 101
Fish, 79-80,83,89
Fitness level, 21-22
Fit or Fat, (Covert Baily) 89
Flexibility, 24,35-36,162
Flourine, 82
Flyes,
    dumbell, 112,118,126
    incline dumbell, 114,126,130,190,194
    incline face-down, 112,172
    pec deck, 112,118,126,131
    supine, 129
Folic acid, 80
Forced negatives, 189
Forearms, 106-121,146,156-157,190
Frequency, 31,104
Fruit, 89
    citrus, 80

G

Gadja, Bob, 193
Gastrocnemius, 39
General sweep, 136
Giant sets, 195
Gironda, Vince, 96

Girth,
    hip, 19
    waist, 19
Glove(s), 70-71
Glutes, 38,135
Glute stretch, 38
Goals, 54,62,104
Good form, 46-47
Goodlad, Elaine, 160
Good mornings, 118,182
Gradual progression, 29
Grains, 83
Grapefruit, 80
Gums, 80
Gym, 72,104
    commercial, 64-67
    home, 64-67
    what to look for in a, 65-67

H

Hack lift(s), 141
Hack machine, 140
Hack squats, 98,140
Halibut, 83
Hamstrings, 38,135,140
Hamstrings stretch, 38
Hanging,
    knee raises, 121,194
    leg raises, 99,163,190,194
Heart, 79
Heartbeat, 202
    regulation of, 82
Heart disease, 19
Heart rate, 30,92
    calculating maximum, 30,92
    target zones of, 30
Heavy and Light Routine, The, 114-115
Heavy duty training, 186
Heel board(s), 72
Heel raise, 98
Height, 20
High blood pressure, 22
High intensity interval training (HIITs), 31,63,116
Hoffman, Bob, 186
Hormone production, 80
Hourglass figure, 176
Human growth hormone, 161
Hydrodensitometry, 19

CREDITS

FRONT COVER PHOTO CREDIT
Paul Buceta
(Hair and Make-up artist – Lori Fabrizio)

BACK COVER PHOTO CREDIT
Paul Buceta
(Hair and Make-up artist – Lori Fabrizio)

INTERIOR PHOTO CREDITS
Cathy Chatterton: pages 8, 81 (*The Eat-Clean Diet Cookbook* cover, **Hair and Make-up artist – Franca Tarullo**), 144

Donna Griffith: page 81
(Food stylist – Marianne Wren)

istockphoto.com: pages 6, 10, 16, 18,19, 21-23, 27, 29, 33-36, 40 (fork and tomato), 41 (skipping rope), 42, 50, 51, 56, 62-65, 67, 68, 70 (dumbell set), 71 (girl with gloves), 74 (multi-purpose bench), 76, 78-80, 82-86, 89, 93, 96,100-102, 122, 126, 134, 146, 160, 161, 176, 188, 189, 194, 202

Paul Buceta (Hair and Make-up artist – Lori Fabrizio): pages 2, 24, 38, 39, 45-47, 52, 70 (training belts), 71 (EZ-curl bar), 72 (Tosca and ankle & wrist weights), 73 (olympic barbell springs), 74 (Tosca and crossover pulley machine), 75 (leg extension machine), 88, 94, 124, 128-131, 136, 137, 140-143, 148-158, 162-166, 168, 170-174, 177-182, 184, 190, 191, 203, 206

Robert Kennedy (Hair and Make-up artist – Franca Tarullo): pages 9, 11, 12, 13, 15, 31, 37, 40, 41, 48, 55, 57, 66, 75 (squat stands), 90, 91, 105, 108, 111, 117, 121, 135, 138, 139, 147, 167, 183, 187, 192, 196, 197, 208, 211, 213, 230

Robert Reiff: pages 73, 123, 127

Terry Goodlad: pages 59, 60, 132, 198, 201

OUTFIT CREDIT
Berns at Passion Fruit Design: pages 38, 39

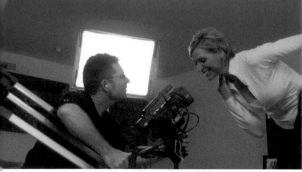
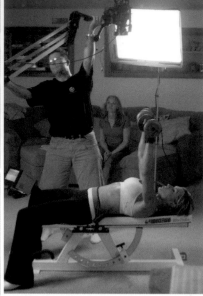
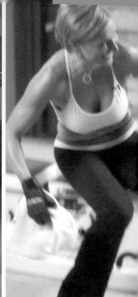
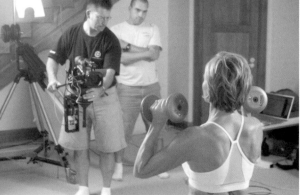
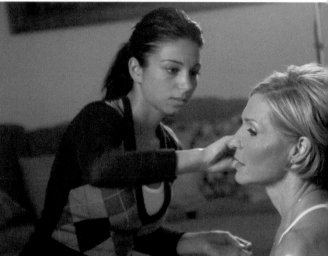
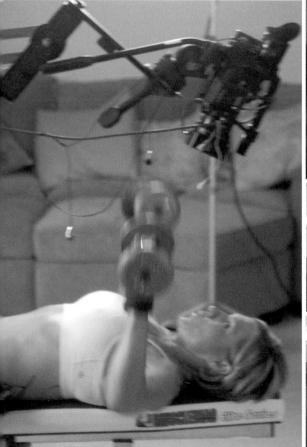
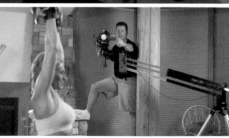
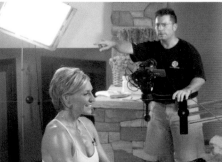
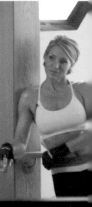

THE DVD SHOOT

ACKNOWLEDGEMENTS

Obviously a book of this magnitude is not created alone. Infinite numbers of people combine to put ink and photo to paper and thus produce a finished product.

Once again I must begin by thanking my husband, Robert Kennedy, a legend in the bodybuilding industry himself, who has handed me the courage and the knowledge to not only believe in myself but sharpened my ability to tell my own story. Many of his images make this book special. Thank you hardly seems enough, but thank you nonetheless.

To my family – a happy mix of brothers, sisters, stepchildren, moms, dads and cousins – who has shouldered me through this journey of mine, I hug and kiss all of you for your love. Rachel, Kiersten, Kelsey-Lynn, Chelsea and Braden you are my children and I love you and thank you for your patience, understanding and support. All of you keep me on the straight and narrow. No Divas allowed!

To the dream team – The Eat-Clean Team , including Wendy Morley and Rachel Corradetti, who craft something magical out of mere words and thoughts. They make the art of bodybuilding come alive in this book. They catch my mistakes, too. Thank you from the bottom of my heart.

To Gabriella Caruso who is undeniably the only person I would ever want to design my books. She has excelled herself and done so in the most professional manner even when the hours were punishing. Gabby your creative touch is divine. Thank you for being you and doing what you do best.

To Paul Bucetta and has photographic team, thank you for your keen eye. You make me look the best I can even when doing squats. Imagine! Thanks to Screaming Monkeys and Coffee Runs, we not only got the job done but we had a blast.

To Mike Sinyi and his video team, I owe a debt of gratitude for your creative eye and persistent demands for more and better footage. You shine on. Even through long hours of filming and editing you kept both your spirit and mine on high. Thank you.

To my makeup talents. Franca, you know what you mean to me. We are friends and we work together like a dream. Thank you for your gift. You are my light. Lori, you make me laugh and you make me look good. What else can a gal ask for? My thanks to you both.

To Berns for creating outfits that suit the woman I am. You are passionate and your fruit shows it. Many thanks.

And to the millions of you who support the Eat-Clean movement. Thanks to you we are going viral. Eating Clean is here to stay.